Psychogeriatrics

An Introduction to the
Psychiatry of Old Age

To Sister Dunsdon and Millie Yates

Psychogeriatrics

AN INTRODUCTION TO THE PSYCHIATRY OF OLD AGE

Brice Pitt MD (Lond), FRCPsych
Consultant Psychiatrist with a special interest in Psychogeriatrics,
The London Hospital;
Recognised Teacher in Psychiatry, University of London

Foreword by
W. Ferguson Anderson
OBE, MD, FRCP
Professor of Geriatric Medicine, University of Glasgow

SECOND EDITION

CHURCHILL LIVINGSTONE
EDINBURGH LONDON MELBOURNE AND NEW YORK 1982

CHURCHILL LIVINGSTONE
Medical Division of Longman Group Limited

Distributed in the United States of America by
Churchill Livingstone Inc., 19 West 44th Street, New
York, N.Y. 10036, and by associated companies,
branches and representatives throughout the world.

First edition 1974
Second edition 1982

ISBN 0 443 01598 8

British Library Cataloguing in Publication Data
Pitt, Brice
    Psychogeriatrics.—2nd ed.
    1. Geriatric psychiatry
    I. Title
    618.97'689   RC451.4.A5

Library of Congress Catalog Card Number 81-69240

Printed in Singapore by
The Print House (Pte) Ltd.

Foreword

Statistical predictions regarding the numbers of older people and their likely disabilities demonstrate clearly the importance of mental disturbances, especially in the very elderly. Thus psychogeriatrics is very relevant to the present development of medical practice and is defined as that branch of psychiatry which is concerned with the whole range of psychological disorders in the over 65 age group.

In this book the subject is covered comprehensively, and while the problems are clearly stated, so also are the solutions. It is well recognised that some 12 per cent of the total population are elderly, but not so well known that one third of those who kill themselves belong to this group, and as the author points out vividly, the type and standard of accommodation frequently offered to elderly mentally ill people leaves much to be desired.

The peculiar way in which man survives for so long after the end of his reproductive life means that losses of many kinds occur and the needs of older people, for example nutrition, warmth, shelter, comfort and cleanliness, are well described. Professional attitudes of defeatism are noted, and the need is rightly stressed for accurate diagnosis. No-one could deny the author's plea for a good psychogeriatric service, and his comment that such work can be exacting but rewarding. The mental diseases of old people are described by a careful classification, and the psychogeriatric service which should meet the needs of the old people in the community is laid down in a most interesting way by comparing the unorganised type of service which often exists, with an effective type; team work, assessment, especially in the patient's home, and liaison are stressed. The need for full co-operation with nurses, social workers, occupational therapists and physiotherapists is emphasised. The rejection of the psychogeriatric patient in the general hospital is noted, but attention is also drawn to the unhappy plight of some elderly mentally ill people in geriatric hospitals where amenity may be of a very poor quality. Dr Pitt, correctly in my opinion, considers that the old person with organic irremedial brain damage is usually better cared for in a psychiatric ward rather than in a geriatric unit.

The very important part played by the patient's family in supporting the elderly mentally ill person at home is stressed. Training of doctors, psychiatrists, nurses, physicians practising geriatric medicine, general practitioners, occupational therapists, physiotherapists and social workers, is also described, as is also the need for more operational research.

The general impression given by this fascinating book is one of optimism. The idea quite clearly stated is that with proper organisation, supporting services which are adequate, and the trained and interested psychiatrist, this is essentially a soluble problem.

Dr Pitt writes in an interesting style which grips the attention, and while the information given is factual and necessary, it is also presented in a delightful and enthusiastic manner.

I benefited greatly from reading this instructive book and I do hope it is widely read. I have no doubt that it will be of immense help to all concerned with the elderly, but perhaps even more important, will immensely improve the care, understanding and prospects of eventual recovery of innumerable elderly people.

Glasgow, 1974   W.F.A.

Preface to the Second Edition

I am glad that the original version of this book is now sufficiently out of date for a second edition to be required. Though not yet fully recognised as a separate specialty within psychiatry, psychogeriatrics and its clientele are here to stay. The great breakthrough since the first edition has been in dementia research, and now a large number of good minds all over the developed world are exercised by this scourge of late life, and hope to discover significant amelioration if not a cure ere long. Such a quest would have been inconceivable only a few years ago when it was widely assumed that dementia was an inevitable part of ageing. Behavioural psychology, too, is starting to show that it can achieve successes in modifying disturbed behaviour in a variety of psychiatric disorders in the elderly just as it can in neurotic younger people and the mentally handicapped. As more and more able clinicians turn to the psychiatry of old age, striving for earlier case finding, more exact diagnosis and more appropriate treatments, a mood of informed optimism, despite many formidable problems, prevails. Economic recessions and reductions in public spending have not prevented the development of a variety of exciting psychogeriatric services in different districts, counties and countries. The bond between psychiatry and geriatric medicine has, happily, been strengthened, and there remains enormous scope for better training for all those who may work with the mentally disordered elderly.

Though I am sure that this remains a thoroughly British book I have been grateful for the opportunity to travel lately in North America and Australia, and have attempted in this edition to make some mention of what happens in other countries. I have been taught much by colleagues at home and abroad and am glad of the opportunity to exploit this in the book. I am relieved too to remove some of the errors to which kindly critics drew my attention after the first edition.

The staff of Churchill Livingstone have been very tactful and persuasive with an occasionally wayward, evasive and overwrought author, and I am grateful to my secretary, Margaret O'Mahoney, who has worked very hard, above and beyond the call of duty, to put the new manuscript together.

London, 1982   B.P.

Preface to the First Edition

I first saw the need for a popular book on the psychiatry of old age in 1967, when I was working with the psychogeriatric firm at Claybury Hospital. I then contacted my present publishers, who showed considerable interest and gave me encouragement. However, I went back into general psychiatry for a spell and only got down to writing the book in early 1973. After this long gestation, the delivery was surprisingly swift and painless and I am grateful to Churchill Livingstone for being such courteous and efficient midwives!

In those seven years since the book's conception, psychogeriatrics as a sub-specialty of psychiatry has developed ever more rapidly, and those few of my colleagues who argue that it should not exist are in no stronger a position than Canute holding back the waves. However, the need for people to work with the mentally disordered elderly is greater than ever, and I hope this primer may possibly attract some to the field, while proving helpful and instructive to those already labouring there.

I must thank my colleagues at The London Hospital, Professor Desmond Pond and Dr Christopher Silver, for their very valuable advice; Drs Tom Arie and Sam Robinson for useful comments; and Professor Ferguson Anderson (whose chairmanship of a 'King's Fund' symposium on Psychogeriatrics I found positively inspiring) for doing me the great honour of writing the foreword.

My thanks are also due to Maureen Marshall and Geraldine Dadd for secretarial services and to the ladies to whom I have dedicated this work, who were with the Claybury psychogeriatric firm from its inception and whose zeal and devotion to their difficult task are models of how to treat psychiatric disorder in the elderly.

London, 1974   B.P.

Contents

1

Psychogeriatrics: the problem

DEFINITION

Psychogeriatrics is an ugly word coined in the early 1960s, when psychiatrists recognised that more and more of their patients were elderly, and geriatricians recognised that they were dealing with large numbers of the confused.

There has not, however, been general agreement about the meaning of the term. Needless to say, it does not refer to deranged geriatricians, or even decrepit psychiatrists! Nor should it be used as the pleural of 'a psychogeriatric', meaning a mentally sick old person: it would be no more appropriate to call a sick child a paediatric! Some people confine 'psychogeriatrics' to the care of the confused and demented elderly, while others apply the word where mental and physical disease occur simultaneously. Most, however, mean by psychogeriatrics the assessment, treatment and management of elderly people suffering all kinds of mental disorder. These include *depression* (which is even more common than *dementia*), *paranoid* states, *neurosis* (mainly manifest as undue *anxiety*) and troublesome quirks loosely labelled *personality* and *behaviour disorders*, as well as acute or chronic states of confusion.

For the purpose of this book, then, *psychogeriatrics* is defined as that branch of psychiatry which is concerned with the whole range of psychological disorder developing in the senium (i.e. after the age of 65). Like a child psychiatrist, the psychogeriatrician is a psychiatrist interested in a particular age group. However, the span covered by his interest is more than 30 years.

THE SIZE OF THE PROBLEM

The older we get, the more liable we are to mental disorder. The number and proportion of old people in every developed country is increasing all the time; in the United Kingdom the percentage of those over 65 has trebled since the beginning of this century.

Therefore the number and proportion of mentally disturbed old people is also increasing, to such an extent that they present the major challenge to the health and welfare services of our society in the closing years of the twentieth century.

Already eight million people in Great Britain (14 per cent are over 65, and more than a third of these are over 75) are the age at which significant disability, mental or physical or both, becomes the rule. According to the Central Office of Information pamphlet *Care of the Elderly in Britain* (1977), by the year 2001 there will have been a 4 per cent increase in those over 65, a 20 per cent increase in those 75–79, a 31 per cent increase in those 80–84, and an increase in those still older of 46 per cent. The elderly would then need three quarters of all the general hospital beds now available for men, and no less than nine tenths of those (excepting maternity beds) for women. Already in most mental hospitals more than half the female patients are over 65. If (as seems not unlikely) many of these hospitals will still function in the twenty-first century they are sure to be used almost entirely for the aged.

Low fertility and a high standard of living have increased the age of the population more than medical advances which lengthen the lives of older people. A hundred years ago it was exceptional to achieve one's 'three score years and ten'. A baby born in Great Britain today, as elsewhere in north west Europe, can be expected to live until at least 70. In the third world there are notably fewer old people (India has barely two or three per cent over 65) though family planning and better public health will certainly soon increase the numbers. Prosperous industrialised Japan stands out from the other Eastern countries with seven per cent of its people aged over 65.

In North America there are not quite so many elderly as in Europe. Ten per cent are over 65 in the United States, under nine per cent in Canada—but the numbers and proportion are growing fast. In the United States the increase in those over 65 since 1900 has been two and a half times as great as in those under that age. In Canada, while the whole population is four times greater than in 1901, those over 65 have increased sevenfold. The elderly population is not evenly distributed within these various countries. In Britain there are areas (the Highlands, for example) which younger people have left in search of work and others, such as the south coast, to which the elderly tend to move on retirement. In Bexhill, Chichester and Worthing, for example, on Britain's 'Costa Geriatrica', those over 65 form more than a third of the total population. The highest proportion of old people in the United States is in

Florida, where the agreeable climate attracts many on retirement and in the winter months. Where there are too few younger people to care for the ailing aged, geriatric and psychogeriatric problems become critical.

In the 50 odd years from the year of my birth, 1931, to the time of my writing this the proportion of middle aged, between 35 and 65, to elderly people has dropped from ten to one to only four to one. Over the same period the proportion of middle aged women, (the chief family supporters of the elderly) going out to work has risen from ten to fifty per cent (Moroney, 1976). So the numbers of potential supporters and their availability have been drastically reduced.

The chance of admission to a psychiatric bed increases sharply in later life, especially for women. The first admission rate to mental hospitals in those over 75 is more than double that in middle life in Britain and one in every four adults admitted to a psychiatric ward is over 65. This may partly reflect the reduced social circumstances of the very old, who tend to be widowed, alone and infirm, and are therefore relatively difficult to care for at home. However, there is abundant evidence from several studies that the prevalence of mental disorder in the elderly at home is very high.

A survey in Newcastle (Kay, Beamish & Roth,1964) showed that 1 in 10 of those over 65 suffered from dementia, and that in half of these the condition was severe. Yet only 1 in 5 of the demented was in an institution of any kind—general, geriatric or psychiatric hospital, or old people's homes; 80 per cent were being looked after —or neglected—at home. Another 15 per cent of those surveyed suffered from depression, anxiety, paranoia or personality disorder of at least moderate severity. Very few were receiving any formal psychiatric treatment and only one in ten was in any kind of institution. When milder conditions were included, altogether 40 per cent of the elderly population were found to be suffering from some form of psychiatric disorder.

From this it seems that the minority of old people in institutions are only the tip of the iceberg. Yet even this minority is felt in some quarters to be bringing the National Health Service to its knees.

It is rarely easy to find a hospital bed for an old person in an emergency. General medical and orthopaedic wards are often more than half filled by the elderly, some of whom stay for months. Many geriatric services are saturated, with dauntingly long waiting lists. Psychiatric hospitals have become increasingly wary of taking in old people whom they may not be able to discharge. Waiting lists for old people's homes, are frequently formidable, and staffs complain that they are having to look after confused and difficult residents without either the inclination or the aptitude to do so. Moans about low morale are, indeed, widespread. It is stated that too many are forced to care for aged patients against their real wishes, and the few who do choose such work are hopelessly overloaded.

Yet there are far more 'out' than 'in', and while many of these are very adequately treated by their doctors, and cared for by their families and the community services, quite a few are not. Mentally disordered old people are much more likely to withdraw than to clamour, and are easily overlooked. They do not often attend doctor's surgeries, and are rarely referred to outpatient clinics (Mezey & Evans, 1971). When a man of 30 stops going out to work, ceases to have sexual relations with his wife and fails to leave his house for 6 weeks on end there will be little difficulty in recognising that something is wrong. But similar behaviour in a man of 70 may well not be noticed, or if it is, may be dismissed with a shrug and the comment 'anno domini'. The sad truth that many old people suffer in silence until too late was surely brought home by the statistics for suicide in 1971: while the elderly constituted 12 per cent of the total population, they formed one third of those who killed themselves.

REFERENCES

Care of the Elderly in Britain 1977 Central Office of Information pamphlet 121. HMSO, London

Kay D W K, Beamish P, Roth 1964 Old age mental disorders in Newcastle-upon-Tyne. Brit J Psychiat 110: 146–158

Mezey G, Evans 1971 Psychiatric in-patients and out-patients in a London Borough. Brit J Psychiat 118: 609–616

Moroney R M 1976 The family and the state: considerations for social policy. Longman, Harlow

2

Ageing and its problems

THE PROCESS OF AGEING

Ageing is the progressive decline in function and performance which accompanies advancing years. It is partly due to a 'wearing out' by accumulated stress and strain, a process which affects inanimate material (e.g. metal fatigue) as well as living organisms. Probably more important, though, is an inborn factor, related to species and sex; elephants, tortoises, parrots and man all live 70 years or more, dogs hardly more than 15, hamsters only 2, and caddis-flies but a single day. In nearly all species the female tends to outlive the male. Women live an average 5 years longer than men and as they tend to be a little younger than the men they marry, there are far more widows than widowers.

The Psalmist says: 'The days of our age are threescore and ten; and though men be so strong that they come to fourscore years, yet is their strength then but labour and sorrow; so soon passeth it away, and we are gone'. This is not merely poetic, but a shrewd clinical observation, for it is after the age of 70 that the effects of ageing are most marked. Interestingly, modern medicine has not greatly increased the life span, but only the numbers of those surviving to be old. At the turn of the century working-class families were very large, and many children died in infancy. Now families are much smaller, but very few children die; indeed, most can expect to live past the age of retirement.

There are various theories about what determines our life span, based mainly upon laboratory studies and animal experiments by gerontologists—biologists with a special interest in ageing. Many of the *cells* which make up the body's organs have to *reproduce* themselves to keep up their number. It used to be believed that small errors in this process would be magnified by successive reproductions; a faulty copy of the DNA (deoxyribonucleic acid) molecules which make up the genes, and have to split up before the cell divides, would lead eventually to cells and organs which could not function properly. Such errors do, indeed, take place, but it is now known that the nucleus of the cells contains a corrective, an enzyme which eliminates the erroneous part of the molecule and ensures a true copy of the correct gene. However, Leonard Hayflick of Stanford University, California, has shown that cells grown outside the body can only reproduce themselves about 50 times; after that they either die out or turn cancerous. This number of doublings is more than enough to see man through the number of years he actually lives now, but sets a limit to the number of years that he could live. It may be that the later cells in the series are less efficient at, say, repairing wear and tear and combatting infection.

Free radicals are very active molecules which contain more or less than the usual number of electrons, or electrons in a high state of energy. Being so active, they very readily combine with other molecules, eventually disrupting or destroying the functions which depend on them. Free radicals cause food to perish, and may contribute to the process of ageing. Radiation increases the number of free radicals and Hiroshima survivors showed some features of premature ageing. Preservatives (antioxidants) are added to foods in cans and jars to stop their perishing, and experiments have been carried out similar substances to see if they slow ageing in mice. They appear to do so, but the interpretation of the results is not easy because those substances may have other effects than reducing the number of free radicals.

For example, as Comfort points out in his heartening book *A Good Age* (1972), if you feed mice a large amount of an unpleasant chemical in their diet they *eat less*. Mice deprived of food on every third day of their lives live almost twice as long as those which enjoy a daily feed. The moral is probably eat less (but don't starve yourself) and live longer.

The connective tissue in which the cells and organs of the body are bedded is subject with ageing to *cross linkage*, whereby large molecules become linked together and the tissue loses some of its qualities. For example, when the long straight hydrocarbon chains of natural rubber become so linked, the rubber loses its elasticity, and a similar process affects the body's form of elastic tissue, collagen. This affects the skin, which becomes more wrinkled with ageing, and the arteries, which become harder. There is a theory that cross linking in DNA could prevent the cell from reading genetic information correctly, and impede the production of necessary enzymes.

The *immune system* of cells and antibodies attacks, neutralises and rejects foreign invaders of the body and is a vital defence against infection. It also rejects grafts of alien tissue into the body, so that it has to be artifically suppressed (at no little risk) for, say, heart and kidney transplants to take. The efficiency of this system dwindles with ageing. Not only are infections resisted less well—influenza can kill a very old person—but the body's ability to recognise itself may be impaired. This is the basis of auto-immune disease, in which the body as it were turns on itself and attacks some of its own tissues. Rheumatoid arthritis and systemic lupus erythematosus are among the acute immune disorders. Various types of auto-antibodies are found more commonly in older people, and it is likely that autoimmunity is an important contributor to ageing.

To quote the Psalms again: 'To everything there is a season, and a time to every purpose under the heaven; a time to be born, and a time to die'.

All life ends in death. Man, however, is aware of this as few, if any, other organisms can be. Man also has, usually, a vivid awareness of himself which makes his own death peculiarly poignant, so from time to time he demands *Why?* and especially *Why me?* But why not? There is almost certainly an evolutionary advantage to a species in replacing its members by reproduction rather than rendering them immortal. Thus death may be seen as the last stage in an inexorable development starting at conception, with birth, growth, maturation, puberty and the menopause important milestones on our journey to the grave. Development and ageing go hand in hand at first, but in later life the ageing process renders us ever more likely to die as we approach the end of our genetically determined life span. The *clock* theory of ageing postulates a programmer, probably located in the hypothalmus in the floor of the brain, which switches these various stages of our lives (and deaths) on (and off) at the appropriate times. The cells of the body may well have their own clocks too, and this may be of particular importance in those, like the nerve cells of the brain, which do not reproduce themselves but have to last us all our lives.

In the course of ageing, the reserve of *adaptation* runs out—like dwindling capital at the bank, or engine oil losing its oiliness. The resources to cope with stresses of all kinds—infections, injury, even moves—diminish. 'Flu can be fatal to the very old, a fractured femur is frequently the final accident, and admission to hospital or an Old People's Home can cause great confusion.

However, people age at different rates. Some are middle-aged at 25, and old at 50, while others retain their youth into their 70s. Heredity plays a part in this, as it does in longevity. So may the amount of stress endured; it seems that those who have suffered prolonged, extreme hardship, e.g. concentration camp survivors, age before their time. Personality and attitudes very probably have their effects too. Cicero observed that old men preserved their intellects if they maintained their interests. Dr Comfort remarks that old people can continue an active sex life well into their seventies and beyond, but often do not because they feel that they will not be able to, or should not anyway at their time of life: he calls this 'bewitchment by expectation'. Loss of the pleasure of sex is therefore less often an effect of true physical ageing than of an attitude to oneself as old and past it!

Nevertheless, ageing of course comes eventually to all who live long enough. The *physical* effects are well known. The *skin* becomes dry, thin and wrinkled, the *hair* white and sparse, the *nails* thickened and brittle. *Bones* lose calcium, and become fragile and bent. Wedging of the softened vertebrae is associated with curvature of the spine. *Muscles* weaken and wither, and *joints* stiffen. The face is less mobile, movements are shaky and the walk is slowed.

There is loss of *hearing* from the 40s onwards: it is normal to be deaf in old age. The deaf old person is particularly liable to be isolated, to be treated with exasperation and even to become morbidly suspicious. *Vision* fails; from the 50s there is difficulty in focusing properly for reading, and in old age actual blindness (due to glaucoma, cataract or degeneration of the retina) is not uncommon. Many old people lose their sense of *smell* and hence most of the pleasures of taste too.

Teeth fall out, the jaw gradually shrinks, and dentures become loose (as all who work with the elderly must know all too well). At the other end of the digestive tract, there is often a troublesome tendency to *constipation*. In men the *prostate gland* enlarges, and sooner or later there is difficulty in passing urine. Old women are extremely liable to *urinary infections*, which undermine their health and contribute to the embarrassing distress of *incontinence*.

The elastic tissues in the body become fibrous, and lose their resilience. This is a factor in lung and heart disease. Also in the *lungs*, the surface area for the exchange of oxygen and carbon dioxide lessens, causing shortness of breath. The loss of elasticity and surface area are commonly associated with *chronic bronchitis*, a crippling disease to which smokers who have spent much of their life working out of doors in towns are especially liable. In the end, of course, many if not most old people succumb to *pneumonia*.

Another important cause of shortness of breath *is heart failure*. *High blood pressure* is one cause of heart failure, and the loss of elasticity in the walls of the *arteries* is one factor in high blood pressure. From middle age onwards arteries are liable to be clogged by *atheroma*, which is responsible for coronary thrombosis and the majority of strokes. Due to atheroma (which particularly afflicts men), the blood supply to various organs is barely adequate at rest, and will fail in an emergency.

Other physical ailments to which the elderly are especially prone include *diabetes, anaemia, cancer, hypothermia* (old people are ill-equipped to withstand the cold to which so many are exposed) and, of course, *accidents*.

Psychologically ageing affects intellect and personality, though how much of this is due to the ageing of the brain and how much to the social aspects of being old is not clear. *Intelligence* tests tend to show that after rising to a plateau in early adult life intelligence dwindles sometime or other after the age of 50, but there is a great deal of variation between individuals. The length and quality of schooling, the motivation of older subjects set tests by and largely designed for younger people, their state of health and the presence of any sensory defects like deafness or impaired vision will all possibly affect performance at intelligence tests without necessarily meaning a loss of basic ability.

Lack of flexibility and creativity may partly be due to lack of alternatives and opportunities as one gets older. Although Sir William Osler's observation that little worthwhile creative work is done after the age of 40 is perhaps generally true (especially of scientists) there are many exceptions! Michaelangelo, Rembrandt, Picasso (and Grandma Moses) all painted vigorously in their seventies and Frank Lloyd Wright designed some of his most exciting buildings in and after his seventieth year. Verdi wrote *Falstaff* in his eighties; De Gaulle, Golda Meir and Bertrand Russell were politically formidable after attaining their three score years and ten; we have a septuagenarian President of the United States in Ronald Reagan; Graham Greene, over seventy, writes novels which continue to fascinate; Ralph Richardson, approaching eighty, has become an incomparable actor of quirky old men; there are so many exceptions to the rule that the rule hardly seems worth stating.

True, older people's *responses* do appear to be *slowed*. This may have something to do with a loss of nerve cells (though we are probably born with far more than we could use in a normal life span) sensory impairment (e.g. poor hearing), slowing of conduction through the nerve fibres, faults in transmission at the synapses between nerves, and delay in the reaction of muscles to nerve impulses. More time is needed for older subjects to match the scores of younger on intelligence tests, and while the knowledge of words is relatively well preserved, new problems are tackled less ably. But experience and knowledge often offset these deficits. In a balanced society, the reflective considered wisdom of the old tempers the impetuous ingenuity of the young.

The well known tendency of old people to remember the remote past more vividly than the recent may in part be because their past *is* more vivid than their present, when life may be very limited and their future short. Octogenarians might be expected to be less concerned about the rate of inflation than those in their twenties, though not a few old people worry about the dwindling value of their capital and the estate they will leave behind them

A distinction has been drawn between the 'normal' forgetfulness of advanced age, and that of dementia (Kral, 1965). The former is regarded as benign, in that nothing is forgotten which really needs to be remembered (e.g. it is necessary to remember where one lives, and that today one collects one's pension, but it does not really matter in the least to most old people who is Prime Minister, or which political party happens to be in power) and while the full details of recent experiences may not be recalled, events are not forgotten in their entirety.

The chief *personality* change is towards greater *introversion*. As the circle of acquaintances contracts and involvement in future plans and even current affairs dwindles, the inner world becomes richer than the outer. A very few intimate companions, even one, suffice. Towards these, in extreme old age, the relationship is one of egocentric, childlike dependency. Habits and routines prevail. There is often a preoccupation with the body's functions, especially the bowels. Sometimes this preoccupation takes the morbid form of hypochondriasis. Reminiscence may be mellow, allowing a broad and philosophical view of life and a tolerant, tranquil view of modern society. On the other hand, the attitude may be peevish and morose: 'change and decay in all around I see'.

It has been said that as we get older we get more 'like ourselves'. Certainly increasing introversion exaggerates certain traits, such as obstinacy, indolence, cantankerousness, miserliness and withdrawal, to the point of caricature. And while one is relatively free to be awkward in earlier life, to be regarded as difficult when one is old and dependent on others is a serious disadvantage (see Ch.11).

LOSSES EXPERIENCED IN OLD AGE

Man (and still more so, woman) is unusual in the animal kingdom in his survival for so many years after the end of his reproductive life. From the *evolutionary* point of view, there must be some advantage. Man is unique both in the richness and complexity of his memory, and in his ability to communicate knowledge to his fellows. Presumably, then, it is for his potential wisdom that he is allowed to survive so long.. Indeed, the Roman senate was largely composed of supposedly wise old men, and hence its name. Even today, it is a positive advantage for a politician, a judge or a fellow of a learned society to be old.

However, the *role* of the elderly in a modern, materialistic, technologically advanced society is not well defined. There are other means of storing information than in the brains of the aged. What else can old people contribute? We seem none too clear.

Occasionally, when hard pressed at work we sigh 'Roll on, retirement' but as the actual time draws near such wishes are expressed with less confidence. Indeed, an attitude very prevalent among the young is 'I hope I never get to be old'. This would seem to bode ill for a phase of life which nearly all will experience.

From the moment of birth, life is marked by *milestones*—critical turning points when we have to give up certain forms of behaviour to take on others. We are bound to regret what we leave behind, but by adopting new attitudes and responsibilities we extend ourselves, and mature as personalities. Weaning, starting school (and later switching to secondary school), puberty, starting work, leaving home, getting married, having children and having them leave home, gaining promotion and facing the menopause are among the most important milestones. Certain birthdays are occasions for 'agonising reappraisal'; while the 21st (or 18th) is usually seen as the 'key of the door' to opportunity and independence, the 30th, 40th and 50th are likely to induce solemn reflections on what has been achieved so far, what may yet be accomplished, and how little time is left.

For some, certain of these milestones are major stumbling blocks. And for many it seems that the greatest of these is that which marks the onset of old age. Ideally, the senium is an opportunity for a final maturation of the personality. The striving, competition and routine drudgery of working years are past, and there is time to pause, consider and take stock. The loss of interest in others, of creativity, the desire to learn, sexual drive, the disengagement from current concerns, which are all supposedly part of normal psychological ageing, favour a state of thoughtful detachment. A few, indeed, seem to reach their prime in old age and glory in their freedom from the tiresome preoccupations and inhibitions of earlier years. 'Grow old along with me' wrote Browning: 'The best is yet to be'.

However, ageing is a period of *decline*. Much must be relinquished, and much endured. It is not given to all to grow old graciously. Losses of all kinds are suffered on a scale which few have experienced before. Some are psychologically unfit to withstand these, while others, through unfortunate (but by no means unusual) circumstances, have more to contend with within a short space of time than anyone could reasonably bear.

The significant *losses* of late life, which contribute directly to the high prevalence of depression at this time, and indirectly to other psychiatric disorders, include those of status, income, health, company, independence, security of accommodation and life itself.

1. Status

Contemporary Western society is materialistic, and spiritual and traditional values count for relatively little. On the whole it is what people do and how much they earn which counts. Old people though accorded the respectful title 'senior citizens', are hardly treated as such. On the contrary, once their working days are over they are seen as dependent members of society with little to offer.

Robert Butler coined the word 'ageism' in 1975 to indicate how older members of the community may be regarded as inferior simply because of their age. While conscious attempts are made to check the harmful and demeaning effects of racism and sexism in most civilised societies, ageism is unfortunately rife. The ageist belittles the needs and importance of the elderly because they have had their life, are no longer productive, can't really appreciate nice things and, being half senile, should not be granted full human rights. The perjorative use of the adjective 'old' is ageist: 'silly old fool'.

However, disregard of the aged may not be a new phenomenon, confined to the western hemisphere or the south of England. Veneration of the elderly in the East may largely have been because of their scarcity value. But Shakespeare's sonnet 'Crabbed age and youth cannot live together', which goes on to declare: 'Age, I do abhor thee; youth, I do adore thee' suggests that antipathy to the old, or 'elder rejection', is not confined to our own times. Families are often accused of not caring about their older members. There are, of course, particular difficulties when children live a long way from their parents, and daughters are under pressure to go out to work. Allowing for this, there is very little evidence that families are less supportive than they ever were, and it is because of their efforts that most infirm old people are still able to survive at home.

Actually the status enjoyed by the elderly varies a good deal with sex and class. In his classic Bethnal Green study Townsend (1957) showed that the working class Nan plays an important role as consultant in child-raising to her daughter, a grandchild minder and a provider of midday meals for her son and son-in-law; even in old age, it seems, 'a woman's work is never done'. Her husband, though, once retired, is utterly unoccupied and in the way, doomed to penury and a life spent on park benches and in public libraries. (Small wonder, then, that sometimes, if his wife falls ill, he finds a purpose in life in looking after her which he may be loth to let go—see Ch.7.) Professional men, on the other hand, are usually able to retire more gradually, and have more leisure interests to pursue. They are houseowners, and have the decoration, repairs and the garden to attend to in their retirement. However, when middle-class couples need their children's assistance they usually have to move some distance to live with or near them, and may be quite at a loss in the new neighbourhood (Wilmott & Young, 1960). Before the era of relatively remote new towns, such as Harlow and Crawley, the extended working-class family tend always to live in the same district and was thus well able to sustain its older members. House-owning old couples may move to the seaside on retirement, which is fine until they become feeble (though even before then they often miss their old haunts and friends). Once they are unable to fend for themselves, however, they are stranded in an area top heavy with old people, and no one who greatly cares to assist them. That important minority who lack family or friends to help them are seen by society as a liability and a burden, a major administration headache, 'the geriatric problem'. And nothing surely reveals the lowly status of our old people than the reluctance of doctors, nurses, social and welfare workers to be professionally responsible for them. It is not that the need is not known; simply, that so few are prepared to meet it.

Perhaps surprisingly there is no statistical evidence that retirement is a significant stress (Richardson, 1965). While for some the loss of occupation is devastating, for others who have been struggling on in poor health from the middle 50s it comes as a great relief.

2. Income

There is often a substantial drop in income following retirement, and most old people have to budget very carefully. Actual poverty is unusual, but there can be few luxuries. The more expensive foods must be avoided, and, unless special rates are made available to pensioners, travel fares are prohibitive. Smokers and drinkers can ill afford to indulge their former habits, which may be good for their health, but not for their happiness. The quality of life, in so far as it is related to money, is reduced.

Pensions are now better related to the cost of living than they were, and some are actually inflation proof, rising annually in line with the rate of inflation. Savings, on the other hand, are not so protected. Inflation is a constant worry to many old people, who cannot strike for more money or put up prices. On the other hand they can vote, and as they form a larger and larger proportion of the community, their power at the polls could become considerable. In the United States, 90 per cent of the elderly are registered to vote. 64 per cent did so in the 1972 presidential election, and 70 per cent in the congressional elections of 1974, compared with only 41 per cent of people between 18 and 24 (Flieger, 1976).

The supplementary pension, a Social Security benefit for those who cannot be expected to live on their state pension alone, helps considerably. However, the supplement is designed to give enough to live on, and no more.

Too many of the elderly, though they should theoretically be able to manage, in fact have sometimes to go cold and hungry and are constantly worried about price rises.

3. Health
The infirmities associated with ageing (listed in the section on The Process of Ageing) cause pain and discomfort, restrict mobility, reduce interaction with the environment and generally impair enjoyment of life. They also lead to increasinng dependency (see (5) below).

4. Company
For many, retirement means the loss of friends who were made and maintained at work. At first this may place considerable strain on the marital relationship. Not every couple who have 'been together now for forty years' still like or love each other very much. Separation is not at all easy for working-class couples with children, and stigma was a deterrent to past generations. They stayed rather unhappily together for convenience, finding welcome distractions from each other at the pub or Bingo hall, but chiefly in work. (Alf Garnett and his wife are an excellent example of this kind of marriage). Then, after retirement, they have to live together, all day. Sometimes they fight, more often they are just unhappy, but not infrequently one or both falls conveniently ill.

This somewhat cynical analysis is not, of course, true of most couples, who are genuinely fond of each other (even though from time to time they get on each other's nerves). For these, as indeed for nearly all who have lived together, even unhappily, for a great many years, the death of one partner subjects the other to the greatest stress of his (or more often her) life. The loss of the most important person in the world, at a time when one is probably less able to adapt than ever before, and exceedingly unlikely to find a substitute, is devastating. It is hardly surprising that, as Murray Parkes has shown, there is a significantly increased risk of the survivor's dying herself or falling seriously ill in the year after bereavement. It is a loss, indeed, from which many old people never recover.

As friends die off there are fewer and fewer with whom the elderly can communicate as peers. True, there are pensioners' clubs, but these seem to cater largely for extroverts, and the less naturally sociable find them hard to use. With reduced means and limited mobility, the task of keeping in touch with a dwindling circle of acquaintance becomes too much. Many will then live essentially alone, and while some are quite content to be so, others are painfully lonely. The highest suicide rate is in elderly men living along.

However, it is possible to feel lonely even when not alone, living for example with one's family, if one has nothing useful to do and nobody to appreciate one's company.

5. Independence
The growing infirmity which ageing brings means increasing dependency on others. This can be quite as painful as the reverse process, whereby the state of dependency is discarded, in adolescence, and the outcome for the personality is more hazardous— destined to be ever more in the hands of others. It takes, indeed, a very mature person to adjust equably to this situation.

Two unhealthy reactions are *denial* and *overanxiety*. Denial is refusal to admit to oneself a painful reality. Denial of dependency involves a failure to recognise serious disabilities, or the need to rely on others. Help is neither sought nor accepted, and there may be stubbornness unto death. Sometimes the community, concerned and somewhat exasperated, pressures its agents into using the law to force these old people into hospital or an old people's home, where they rarely do well. It may be kinder, if reasoning and persuasion fail, to allow them to deteriorate slowly and pass away at least in peace.

Overanxiety is displayed by those who have always needed in

their relationships reassurance that they are effective, serviceable and worth-while. Ageing and the threat of dependency cause a decline in self-confidence and self-esteem. A frightening sense of weakness leads to what Goldfarb (1965) describes as a 'search for aid' from someone seen as strong—the spouse, one of the children, a neighbour, very often the doctor—towards whom the anxious person acts like a helpless child seeking the attentions of a powerful parent. Unfortunately the fear of rejection is so great that clamorous, premature demands are made which tend to alienate the person whose help is so desperately wanted, bringing about the very rejection which is dreaded. For example, the clinging old lady who keeps bringing her daughter to her side by phoning to say that she dying may be felt to have cried 'Wolf!' once too often, and the agitated hypochondriac may exhaust her general practitioner's patience and be consigned to the outpatient departments of various hospitals for an endless series of investigations.

In contrast, Goldfarb says, mature old people, though grieved and shaken by loss and decline, still want and are capable of self-assertion, and a measure of control over their surroundings and their fate. Throughout their lives they have taken pleasure with and not through others.

6. Accommodation

Too many old people live in thoroughly unsuitable accommodation, old, dingy, cluttered, ill-lit, on various levels and with an outside toilet—only ideal, one might think, for falling and freezing in. However, it is home, and rehousing is for some a stress comparable to bereavement. In new and more luxurious surroundings they feel lost, and forlorn. In a tower block some former slum-dwellers feel very isolated, and particularly miss having a front door at street-level. Old people's homes best suit the more compliant, dependent and infirm. Others chafe at the necessary restrictions, loss of privacy and the lack of a front door to call their own. Old people who are not sick but merely infirm are sometimes misplaced in hospital, where life is still more restricting. However, they may be reluctant to commit themselves to an old people's home, for while in hospital they can be looked after, yet keep open the option, however illusory, of return to a place of their own. Old people who have moved in with their families, in two or three generation households, sometimes feel and are felt to be in the way. The arrangement whereby the aged parent lives by turn with each of his children didn't work for King Lear (see Shakespeare) and rarely turns out well.

7. Life

We are, of course, all mortal, but cannot usually bear to be aware of the fact for very much of the time. Death was much more familiar to past generations, when infectious diseases carried off so many so young, and religion played a major part in focusing attention on the hereafter. Now our society is largely irreligious, death is mainly confined to old age, and 'denial' of the fact of dying may contribute to the previously mentioned phenomenon of 'elder rejection,' or not wanting to know about the old.

Despite the nearness of death, I have not found that elderly psychiatric patients are any readier for it than the young. In group discussions, where not infrequently a participant of the previous week has died, the subject seems to be taboo. Yet a reality so imminent and so final can hardly be wholly ignored, and if not faced and come to terms with must surely add to the distress of being old.

For some suggestions about the alleviation of loss in old age see Chapter 13.

THE NEEDS OF THE ELDERLY

The basic needs of the elderly are much the same as those of people generally. However, as it cannot be taken for granted that they will all be met, it is as well to spell them out.

The basic *physical* needs are nutrition, warmth, shelter, comfort and cleanliness.

Nutrition may be inadequate for a variety of reasons, including food fads, ignorance of dietary needs, poverty, infirmity, absent or ill-fitting dentures. 'Infirmity' includes those too feeble to shop, cook, or feed themselves, too confused to know what they are doing, too depressed to care, or preferring alcohol to food. Malnutrition is a cause as well as an effect of ill-health in old age, most often taking the form of *anaemia* due to lack of iron or folic acid. The picture of serious vitamin deficiency is fortunately much less common.

The provision of home helps and Meals on Wheels to the infirm elderly at home does much to prevent serious malnutrition. Indeed, these may be regarded as the twin pillars of the domiciliary services. Remarkably, Meals on Wheels in Britain are for the most part provided by a voluntary organisation—the Women's Royal Voluntary Service. Meals are clean, appetising and served warm in the home, but in most areas are not available to the individual more than two or three times a week. Often, though, there is a local luncheon club where those who can make their way there will get a similar meal on other days.

In institutions nutrition is generally well catered for, though there are obviously difficulties in ensuring that the food which the patient or resident actually eats is as nourishing as that bought on his behalf. Some years ago there was evidence that the diet consumed by the patient in some mental hospitals was deficient in Vitamin C (Leitner & Church, 1956): a recent dietary assessment of a small sample of demented patients in the London Hospital (St Clement's) also showed a deficient intake of Vitamin C (and of folate). These deficiencies were attributable to a lack of fresh fruit, the small quantities of vegetables consumed, and the methods of cooking the vegetables. A salutary paper by Davies & Holdsworth (1979) listed 26 nutritional 'at risk' factors in residential homes for the elderly. These included a lack of rapport with the cook, failure to let residents choose the size of their portions or second helpings, no facilities to provide their own food or drink, poor presentation of food, rushed meals, insufficient help in feeding frail residents, and food 'perks' of staff to the detriment of patient's meals! It is to be hoped that this somewhat Dickensian picture is uncharacteristic, but it cannot be said to be a complete caricature. Where kitchens are far removed from the dining-areas, food may lose some of its quality during the delay between its being cooked and eaten. But the biggest and most deplorable problem is where there are too few staff to see that old people who cannot feed themselves get enough to eat. Here a policy of 'open visiting' pays dividends, for interested relatives may be able to give staff invaluable help at mealtimes.

No discussion of nutrition would be complete without a mention of *obesity*. As we get older we do less and require fewer calories. The failure to modify food intake accordingly is responsible for the 'middle-aged spread'. Also, food may become a substitute for other pleasures, less available once youth has faded. Carbohydrates, such as bread, potatoes and confectionery, are filling, fairly cheap and appeal to those with a sweet tooth; they are, however, very fattening. Life insurance companies know very well that over-weight reduces life expectancy. It is also associated with a great deal of disability: diabetes, arthritis, high blood pressure and heart disease in particular. The obese elderly patient has particular difficulty in getting about.

A diet which drastically reduces carbohydrates, while allowing as much in the way of protein and fat as the patient fancies and providing adequate vitamins, will soon bring weight down to the level appropriate to her age and height. If she is at home, the biggest obstacle is likely to be psychological resistance, and she may need a lot of persuasion and support to give up present comforts for future benefits. In institutions a sentimental attitude by some of the staff can be a handicap. Many, well-meaning, are all to ready to fill up their 'old dears' with sweet tea, cakes, bread and jam. Indeed, obesity is one of the hazards of institutional life-the result of over-feeding and underactivity. All staff must appreciate that diets are to be taken seriously, and that sometimes misguided kindness can kill.

We cannot take it for granted that our old people are *warm* enough, for too many are admitted to hospital (and others die at home) with *hypothermia*. This clinical term (which literally means 'having too low a temperature') is a euphemism for freezing to death. The ordinary clinical thermometer does not read low enough to indicate the true state of hypothermia, when the temperature may be less than 32° Centigrade (90° Fahrenheit). An underactive thyroid conduces to hypothermia, but the reason most often is the combination of cold weather and an inadequately heated home, and while the condition continues the public conscience deserves no ease. Meanwhile, every ward admitting the elderly requires a special low-reading thermometer.

Two large-scale surveys of body temperatures in elderly people living at home were carried out in the winter of 1972. Most of the homes visited were cold with room temperatures below the minimum recommended by the Department of Health. Deep body temperatures below 35.5°C were found in 10 per cent of those studied who were, therefore, at risk of developing hypothermia (Fox et al, 1973).

Very few old people in the West lack *shelter*, though the quality of the roof over their heads often leaves something to be desired. The spectacle of the aged living in the streets, commonplace in the East, is happily rare here, and there are not many over 65 years of age among the pathetic band of our homeless. However, whether at home or in hospital, too often old people tend to occupy the oldest and most derelict accommodation. The typical geriatric ward in Britain is in an indifferently upgraded workhouse, and psychiatric wards for the elderly were for a long time among the most crowded and neglected in the mental hospital. The awfulness of the sanitary annexes to some psychogeriatric wards was staggering. They were damp, encrusted with lime, smelly and bitterly cold. It might be considered, under these circumstances, that the saner patients would wet themselves in the warm. It is ironical that the worst hospital accommodation should have been reserved for those who stay in hospital longest; most admission and short-stay wards are perfectly habitable. It might be thought that old people get the worst accommodation because they are least likely to protest.

However, since this book was first published in 1974 there have been improvements. Scandals arising from the poor quality of institutional care have pricked the public conscience and created a demand for better care for old people (often voiced by community health councils) to which government has responded. In England the Department of Health and Social Services has issued guidance and discussion papers (e.g. *A Happier Old Age*, 1978) and has attempted to safeguard the interests of the elderly and the mentally ill in a period of 'negative growth' and reallocation of resurces in an indigent health service precariously financed by a failing economy (*The Priorities Document*, 1976). Consequently the right of geriatric and psychogeriatric patients to a place in the district general hospital has been conceded and in the north west of England at least there have actually been built brand new psychogeriatric units.The Health Advisory Service surveys geriatric and psychiatric services up and down the country, and though without the powers of an inspectorate, offers constructive criticism and tries to encourage good practice. The Royal College of Nursing and the British Geriatric Society (1975) have jointly issued guidance or minimum standards to be maintained in the care of old people in hospital.

Conditions in the homes provided by the local authorities and voluntary bodies in Britain have improved immeasurably since the middle 1960s. Many have been especially built for old people, while others are converted country houses. The dreadful old workhouses, such as Southern Grove Lodge in Bow, so well described by Townsend in *The Last Refuge* (1962) have been almost entirely abandoned. The only snag is that too few are placed near shopping centres or other local amenities. In the United States the Joint Information Service of the Americal Psychiatric and Mental Health Associations made a fairly favourable report on nursing homes in 1976, and the Office for Nursing Home Affairs aims to improve standards.

Comfort and cleanliness are less vital than the foregoing, but the cheerlessness of so many old people's lives is distressing. Comforts taken for granted in an affluent society may not be theirs. For example, it is a pity that few can afford a telephone, with which to keep in touch with family and friends, or television, to while away the empty hours. It is particularly sad when pets are not allowed to council tenants. (I was asked to see a supposedly confused old lady who talked to an imaginary budgerigar: it turned out that the bird was quite real, but the old lady was cute enough not to let the council know!) Elderly people in hospital and homes need some personal possessions and clothing and a place in which to keep them.

Cleanliness may be next to godliness, but plenty of old people seem to manage quite well without either. Some lack a bathroom, or are too arthritic to get into a bath. A district nurse may help here, though one doesn't need an SRN to wash down an old lady, and some local authorities wisely employ special 'bathers' for the purpose. When demoralised one ceases to care about appearances or hygiene, and this may be a sign of depression. Then there is a small group of eccentric old people who seem to relish living in filth (see the *senile squalor syndrome*, Ch.11). Incidentally it always astonishes me when old couples, who see no one except each other from one month's end to the next, are found to be lousy, I almost doubt the theory of evolution, and reconsider that of spontaneous generation!

Among the basic *psychological* needs are respect, security and self determination.

Respect for oneself needs to be reinforced by respect from others. Those who deal with the elderly should not address them as 'Gran', 'Pop' or 'Dear', nor use their first names unless invited to do so, but give their surname and title.

Majorie Fry wrote: 'To the administrator an individual may be just "that old woman-I think her name is Jones'. But to herself she is the Katie Jones who won a prize for scripture and had the small est waist in the class, with a thousand other distinctive features, who just happens to be old'. We should try to think of our client or patient as a person with a past who has become old but still has something to contribute, if only reminiscences (and how fascinating and enlightening these reminiscences can be, if only we will take time to listen to them), and not just just as an old soul who presents a problem.

The *security* old people need is a reasonable expectation of continuing care, of help when needed, as a right and not a favour, and of not being pushed from pillar to post without warning or consultation. It is frighteningly easy to deny the elderly their rights as human beings and take drastic decisions 'for their own good' without their knowledge or consent. The important subject of civil liberty in old age is most ably discussed in the National Corporation for the Care of Old People's book *Rights and Risk* (1980). In institutions we should see that old people retain their glasses, false teeth and hearing aids and have access to some of their own clothes, however difficult this may be; otherwise, we are taking away their personalities to turn them into merely patients. We should never move them to another ward, hospital or home without prior notice—yet how often, in practice, is this given?

Self-determination, when one is in fact dependent on others, must be limited. However, when there is the possibility of choice, if only about which vegetable or sweet to have, it should be given. Institutions for the elderly should be flexible enough to allow their inhabitants some freedom to decide how to spend their day—what to wear, where to go, what to do, where to sit, when to go to bed—at the very least.

REFERENCES

British Geriatrics Society and Royal College of Nursing 1975 Improving geriatric care in hospital. Royal College of Nursing, London

Butler (1975) Why survive? Being old in America! Harper and Row, New York

Comfort A (1977) A good age. Mitchell Beazley, London

Comfort A (1979) The biology of senescence, 3rd edn. Churchill Livingstone, Edinburgh

Davies L, Holdsworth D (1979) A technique for assessing nutritional 'at risk' factors in a residential home for the elderly. Journal of Human Nutrition 33: 165

Department of Health & Social Security (1976) Priorities for health & personal social services in England. HMSO, London

Department of Health & Social Security (1978) A happier old age. HMSO, London

Flieger H (1976) We're showing our age. US News and World Report 80(8): 20

Fox R H Woodward, P M, Exton Smith A M, Green M F, Donnison D V, Wicks M H 1973 Body temperatures in the elderly: a national study of physiological, social and environmental conditions. Brit Med J 1: 200-206

Glasscote R, Beigel A, Butterfield A Jr, Clark E, Cox B, Elpers R, Gudeman J E, Lewis R, Miles D, Raybin J, Reifler C, Vito E 1976 Old folks homes. J I S of the APA, Washington

Goldfarb A I 1965 The recognition and therapeutic use of the patient's search for aid. In: Psychiatric disorders in the aged. W P A Symposium. Geigy, Manchester

Kral V A 1965 The senile amnestic syndrome. In Psychiatric disorders in the aged. W P A Symposium. Geigy, Manchester

Leitner Z A, Church I C 1956 Nutritional studies in a mental hospital. Lancet 1: 565–567

Norman A, 1980 Rights and risk; a discussion document on civil liberty in old age. National Corporation for the Care of Old People, London

Parkes C M 1965 Bereavement and mental illness. Brit J Med Psychol 38: 1

Richardson I M 1965 Retirement and health. In: Psychiatric disorders in the aged. W P A Symposium. Geigy, Manchester

Townsend 1957 The family life of old people. Routledge and Kegan Paul, London. Penguin, Harmondsworth

Townsend 1962 The last refuge. A survey of residential institutions and homes for the aged in England and Wales. Routledge and Kegan Paul, London

Willmott P, Young M 1960 Family and class in a London suburb. Routledge and Kegan Paul, London. Penguin, Harmondsworth

3

Professional attitudes

Unhappily, work in the field of psychogeriatrics is often impeded by the attitudes of those who have to undertake it. These harmful ageist prejudices need to be identified in order to be recognised and avoided. Chief among them are defeatism, domination and insularity.

Defeatism regards illness in the elderly as the inevitable consequence of their age, and therefore chronic and insoluble: 'You're not as young as you were, you know. 73? What can you expect at your age?'

Doctors with this outlook are obsessed with the notion that brain disease colours all mental illness in those over 65, and to this they ascribe their therapeutic failures. The 'anno domini' philosophy totally disregards those old people who live full, active lives into their 80s and even 90s. Treatment is withheld until there is a crisis, when custodial care, anywhere, is demanded. The resources for such care are inadequate, and tend therefore to be misused, sick people being admitted to old people's homes, or the wrong sort of hospital (psychiatric rather than general or geriatric, and vice versa) and social problems relieved by admission to acute medical and surgical wards, whence the indignant cry soon goes up for 'disposal'!

This attitude causes work with the aged to be regarded as inferior to that with younger, a third-rate occupation for those who cannot find any better employment. (Some colleagues used to regard me as a saint, ill-used, washed up or just plain crazy!) Two recent pieces in the popular medical journal *World Medicine*, one entitled *Geriatric cuckoo* (in the general hospital nest), the other *The myth of geriatrics?* (a 'dud' specialty) show all too plainly the prejudice against old people who 'block' valuable acute beds, and against geriatricians. The American Group for the Advancement of Psychiatry (1971) listed negative staff attitudes towards treating the elderly which no one could reasonably condone and Brooke (1973) found that many psychiatrists in training indicated that they would rather emigrate than practise psychogeriatrics. It is to be hoped that they have been better taught since then, for their services are very much needed in a branch of psychiatry which they could and should find extremely worthwhile. Already one in ten psychiatrists for adults in Britain declares a special interest in the elderly, but more than twice that number is needed. It is not the nature of the work, but simply the defeatist attitude of so many professions to it, which discourages recruitment.

Domination takes two forms. The first—a hostile, *disparaging*, authoritarian attitude—is the more obvious. It arises, perhaps, from frustrated 'omnipotence'. Many of those in the healing professions have a deep need to see their patients get better. Otherwise they feel anxious and unhappy and doubt their own worth. Such doctors and nurses make terrible patients, and they do not adjust too well to old age either. When faced by the difficult problems of their elderly patients they feel helpless, angry and, presumably, an uncomfortable identification with their charges — 'there, despite the grace of God, go I in the not too distant future'. They react by denial and rejection, referring contemptuously to 'those geriatrics' as if they were another species. Such people do not make the best use of their resources, and set a very bad example to their juniors. They could not be helped to find old people less threatening without a fundamental change in their personality, and so are much better employed in treating those with whom they feel more at ease. Unfortunately staff shortages are often such that they cannot be spared to do so.

The other, subtler, form of domination is by an excessively *sentimental* patronising approach: 'They're just like children, really. Isn't she a sweet old duck?' Though well-meaning, this attitude, like the former, robs the elderly client or patient of her dignity, and exaggerates dependence. It, too, may spring from an anxious over-identification with the patient's vulnerability and mortality, leading to a misguided 'doing-as-I-would-be-done-by'. I recall a very nice matron of an old people's home who treated her residents rather as Snow White did the Seven Dwarfs, and saw that they all hung out their stockings on Christmas Eve, apparently under the impression that 'second childhood' had restored their belief in Santa Claus. Another devoted nurse, sister on a supposed rehabilitation on ward, tucked in all her 'old dears' in at night, with a kiss, and was there to wake them with a cup of tea every morning. She pampered and protected them and under her care they were fat, slothful, unenterprising but very appreciative. It was only after her departure and the introduction of a more vigorous regime which required more of them that they were revealed as selfish, bitchy and unreasonable like the rest of us. As they did so they became far more active and started at last to leave hospital.

Old people far too easily fall victims to their attendant's emotional needs.

With the best intentions the Royal College of Nursing's campaign to improve the image of geriatric nursing could have the opposite effect. A robust, apparently alert old lady is shown walking with a frame. *Geriatrics*, reads the poster, *what can we do to help* **them?**. This makes them sound like old donkeys out to grass or whales in need of protection, not out older, frailer selves.

Insularity in the practice of psychogeriatrics means performing one's duty, as one sees it, without reference to any of the other workers who might be involved. In the United Kingdom, health service workers may approach the old person from the primary health care team, or the hospital, and there is an unfortunate division between health and social services. Within each there are a number of different workers who can be involved with an old person at home; the general practitioner, health visitor, district nurse, home help, Meals on Wheels provider, the local geriatrician, psychiatrist, and social workers from the hospital and from the local authority could easily all visit within the course of a few days, many doing so without realising that the others had called in too. A neighbour, a member of the family, a friend, the priest and various voluntary workers could also be in attendance.

At first sight this richness and diversity of personnel may seem impressive, but proper communication between so many different people is difficult, and requires effort and goodwill. Without it, however, the scope for reduplication of effort, demarcation disputes, buck-passing, back-biting and blaming is great. Regular meetings of all those involved in the field are essential to make sure that the ground is properly covered. It helps, too, if people are prepared not to regard their roles too rigidly.

Properly practised, psychogeriatrics is deeply rewarding. The psychiatrist finds that he is fully extended, and that none of the skills he has acquired during his training are superflous. His basic grounding in medicine is needed more than in other branches of psychiatry. He also requires a good understanding of social medicine, and a grasp of family psychodynamics strictly comparable to that necessary in child psychiatry. He and his team must acquire the special rehabilitative skills of the geriatrician, who has probably done more than any other member of the medical profession to get the bedridden up and reduce chronicity in hospitals. The psychogeriatrician should attend autopsies, and see that they are performed, so that he can check his clinical diagnosis. He should know enough about psychological testing, electroencephalography and other neurological investigations to ask for them appropriately and make sense of the results.

Above all, he needs clinical acumen. He has a wider range of disorders to deal with than are shown by younger patients, and a multiplicity of causes. He must evaluate confusion, remembering that what has developed recently and acutely is likely to prove reversible, provided, firstly, that the cause is sought and found or, secondly, that nothing is done in the way of hasty admission to hospital or Old People's Home, relegation to a chronic ward or overmedication, to complicate the issue with a process that is irreversible. He must distinguish between what is relevant, and what incidental. He must strive to find out, from whatever sources he can tap, as much as possible about patients who are deaf, muddled or unable to express themselves (dysphasic). He will not rely all that much on textbook descriptions, because typical pictures of psychiatric disorder are relatively unusual in the elderly. He will not be afraid to treat energetically, wherever appropriate, using the full range of therapy from leucotomy and ECT to psychotherapy. However, he will not feel under a compulsion to treat what is untreatable, or better left alone, for the sake of doing something. He will accept the limitations of a one-man band, and work within a psychogeriatric team, consisting of doctors, nurses, social workers, occupational therapists, physiotherapists and psychologists. All within the team should respect the skills, attitudes and special difficulties of the other members. All need to come to terms with their own feelings about ageing, dependency and death.

The usual effects of the introduction of a psychogeriatric 'firm' (Arie, 1971; Godber, 1978) are to increase admission rate, turnover, discharges, referrals and staffing and reduce deaths, beds and the numbers on the waiting list. Domiciliary visiting, community psychogeriatric nursing and day hospital places are also likely to increase. There is thus a more intensive use of fewer beds and a much greater emphasis on work in the community.

SUMMARY

1. There is a crying need for good psychogeriatric services to the community, and the chief goal of these is to provide assessment, treatment and support for the elderly at home, rather than custodial care.

2. Psychogeriatrics can be exciting and rewarding.

REFERENCES

Allen C 1980 The myth of geriatrics? World Medicine: 11
Arie T 1971 Morale and the planning of psychogeriatric services. Brit Med J 3: 166
Brooke P 1973 Psychiatrists in training. Brit J Psychiat, Special Publication No 7.
  Headley, Ashford
Godber C 1978 Conflict and collaboration between geriatric medicine and
  psychiatry. In: Isaacs B (ed.) Recent advances in geriatric medicine. Churchill
  Livingstone, Edinburgh
Lawrence M 1979 Geriatric cuckoo. World Medicine: 19
Wattis J, Wattis L, Arie T 1981 Psychogeriatrics: a national survey of a new branch
  of psychiatry. Brit Med J 1: 1529

FURTHER READING

Leeming J T (ed.) 1976 Doctors and old age. British Geriatrics Society, Surrey
British Medical Journal 1981 The future of cardiology and psychogeriatrics. Brit
  Med J 283: correspondence, 377, 494–496, 671–672, 791

4

Classification of psychiatric disorders in the elderly

The disorders with which psychogeriatrics is concerned are classified thus:

1. Mental illnesses
   a. Organic
      (i) Delirium (acute confusional state)
      (ii) Dementia (chronic confusional state)
   b. Functional
      (i) Affective illness: depression; mania
      (ii) Paranoid states
      (iii) Neuroses
2. Personality and behaviour disorders

Psychiatric disorders cannot be classified as precisely as physical disorders because the causes are less well known. The division between 'mental illnesses' and 'personality and behaviour disorder' indicates that the former are abnormal states of mind causing a person to be different from his former self, whereas the latter represent long-standing personality traits which have become troublesome at the time of ageing, or vagaries of behaviour not associated with a change in the total personality. The distinction between 'organic' and 'functional' mental illnesses is a causal one, as the 'organic' group are known to be the consequence of brain disease, while the 'functional' are not. However, the subsequent grouping relies mainly on description of the most striking feature of the illness, without in any way suggesting how it developed.

Labels like these are useful in showing the general nature of a disorder, how it differs from others, how it is likely to develop and in providing a basis for teaching and study. For instance, 'depression' means that the patient is suffering from a disturbance of mood not known to be the direct result of brain disease, rendering him abnormally miserable but not impairing his intellect. 'Dementia', on the other hand, means a loss of intellectual ability (of which one of the most obvious signs is a very bad memory) due to permanent and usually progressive brain disease, to which any emotional disturbance is likely to be secondary. Study of groups of patients suffering from each of these disorders has shown that they are distinct, and run a different course. Depression has a natural tendency to recovery (and its duration can be shortened by various treatments) while dementia rarely improves, but on the contrary gets worse and ends in death after a few years or less. In the following chapters I shall deal seperately with these disorders and the others listed at the head of this chapter.

However while these conditions can exist in 'pure' form, in real life they rarely do so. Doctors are taught to try to explain all their findings in a sick person by a single disease process, but such elegant diagnosis is not often possible in the elderly, and the ingenuity required is likely to involve considerable distortion. It is the rule for the very old to suffer several different maladies at the same time, physical as well as mental, some the consequence of others, and some quite separate. A man of 70 referred to me was, according to his doctor, afflicted by diabetes, high blood pressure, ischaemic heart disease, an old stroke, arthritis, prostatic enlargement and cataracts. (All the same, he was well able to walk about.) He had been thought to be manic-depressive in the past, was sometimes confused (presumably because the blood supply to his brain was impaired by atheroma) and lately had been very paranoid towards his wife, which was why I was asked to see him. In hospital most of these diagnoses were confirmed (though we were not too sure about the manic-depression), but his diabetes was very hard to control; the reason, it turned out, was that he also had pulmonary tuberculosis!

The presence of one psychiatric disorder does not rule out the possibility of another. Also, a diagnostic label is useful as far as it goes, but that is not very far. Depressives and demented patients differ among themselves as much as people do in general. Personality is paramount, often determining whether an illness occurs at all, colouring the clinical picture and materially modifying the outcome. So, in psychiatry, we incorporate the diagnosis into a formulation, or brief historical statement of the constitution, the personality and the stresses, past and present, all of which many have contributed to the development of this particular kind of reaction at this time.

5

Delirium (or acute confusional state)

Most people's idea of delirium is probably based on the dramatic delirium tremens (DTs) suffered by alcoholics, either suffering a nightmarish *Lost Weekend* (like Ray Milland in the famous film), haunted by creepy-crawlies, or genially besotted but troubled by the spectacle of pink elephants.

Usually, though, delirium takes a milder form, to which those whose brain is immature or imperfectly functioning are particularly liable. Children in the throes of a fever commonly wake at night, unnaturally bright and chatter on in a way which suggests that they are enacting a waking dream, seeing and talking to imaginary people and misperceiving the real-life situation. Similarly, old people are readily rendered delirious by a wide variety of stresses, mainly but not exclusively physical, which impair the brain's performance. Those old people in whom the blood supply to the brain has become precarious because of clogging by atheroma are particularly susceptible to delirium. For reasons which are neither clear nor very logical the term 'acute (or subacute) confusional state' is generally preferred to 'delirium' where the elderly are concerned.

The onset is fairly sudden, leading from normality to gross disturbance in the course of a day or two. *Confusion*, the cardinal sign of organic mental illness, is always present, but the severity fluctuates. This confusion comprises *impairment of memory*, especially for very recent events (most patients who recover recall little or nothing of their delirium) and *disorientation* so that the patient may not know where he is, the time of day or those about him. Typically confusion is most marked in the evening, when the light is starting to fail and the surroundings are less readily perceived. *Thinking* is disturbed, and comprehension and reasoning are faulty. There is a failure to grasp basic information about the situation and circumstances; a state of muddled perplexity is typical. Talk may be slowed or accelerated, but is almost always disjointed, and the point of all but the simplest and briefest utterances is soon lost.

Disordered *wakefulness* is a cardinal feature of delirium (Lipowski, 1980), manifest as drowsiness (clouding of consciousness) sleeplessness, vivid dreams or heightened alertness. In the course of the day, or even within a few minutes, there may be variations from a state approaching lucidity to one of babbling incoherence. *Concentration* is exceedingly limited: the patient's attention is hard to gain and harder to keep, partly because of marked distractibility.

The mood is *labile,* a dreamy, dazed state changing with disconcerting suddenness to one of fear, anger, excitement, suspicion or perplexity.

Although seriously ill, the patient *cannot rest* for long, but tosses and turns, throwing off the bedclothes or, when even more seriously ill, merely plucks at them and sleeps only in snatches, often being more wakeful at night than by day. Sometimes he will roam the house or ward, searching, miming familar actions (e.g. sewing, drawing curtains) or seeking a way out.

Misinterpretations are common. People are misidentified, and their actions misunderstood, which can form the basis of delusions. *Illusions* occur (i.e. false perceptions), usually visual and promoted by poor lighting and strange sounds. For example, the pattern of wall-paper may be seen as a swarm of cockroaches on the move, the fluff on a blanket can look like the waving fronds of a fungus, or the low voice of a nurse giving the night-report might be heard as plotting or a threat.

Hallucinations occur, i.e. perceptions without an outside stimulus—seeing shapes or hearing voices which are not there—and again, these are mainly visual, which is characteristic of organic disorders. They happen most often when the patient is least awake, or even actually asleep, for hallucinations can follow a nightmare after the patient has woken.

Delusions (firmly held false beliefs arising in the course of mental illness) are common, and almost always *paranoid,* the patient believing himself to be persecuted and victimised. (There is a marvellous account of these in Evelyn Waugh's semi-autobiographical *The Ordeal of Gilbert Pinfold.*) Usually the delusions are transient and vague, but they can be the basis of bouts of aggressive and disturbed behaviour.

Physically the patient is almost always ill—seriously so in the most acute states. There is a rapid pulse, often a fever, dehydration (a dry tongue, sunken eyes and inelastic skin) and the hands shake (hence the 'tremens' in DTs). There are also the more specific signs of the illness underlying the delirium.

In comparison with younger patients, delirium in the elderly is more easily provoked, less dramatic and the symptoms can last longer—occasionally even for weeks. This subacute form can be most perplexing, as the physical basis may not be at all obvious.

The course of delirium is that of the underlying disease. Usually it ends, in full recovery or death, within a week or two. Very occasionally, though, it is followed by dementia.

Delirium, like fever, is a manifestation of a toxic process affecting the whole body and interfering with the brain's activity in various ways—by reducing the oxygen available to the cells, their supply of glucose, flooding them with toxins, inhibiting their enzymes, depriving them of water and upsetting the balance of electrolytes. An imbalance of the neurotransmitters, such as noradrenaline, serotonin and acetyl choline, by which impulses are passed from one nerve cell to the next is also likely. These conditions will now be considered in a little detail, as they well illustrate the diversity of stresses which can confuse the elderly.

1. *Infection*, especially of the lungs; the elderly chronic bronchitic can easily develop pneumonia, of which at first there may be few other signs, not even fever, than his confusion. Cellulitis (acute inflammation of the skin and underlying tissues) is also often associated with delirium in the very old. Urinary infection is very common in old age, and when severe may contribute to confusion.

2. *Cerebral hypoxia* (an abnormally low level of oxygen in the brain), due to:

a. Poor *blood supply* to the brain, mainly because of atherosclerosis—clogging of the arteries with atheroma (the waxy deposit, formed from cholesterol, which also causes coronary thrombosis) and thickening and hardening of their walls. Atheroscleroris is the commonest basis of acute confusional states (followed by pneumonia). The sudden obliteration of an artery serving a sizeable area of the brain's surface is followed by confusion for a few days or several weeks, until the circulation has been restored. A succession of these episodes, separated by intervals of weeks, months or more than a year, may end in a major stroke, or the development of dementia (see Ch. 6). Sometimes a similar effect is produced by occlusion of the major arteries supplying the cranium—the internal carotid and vertebral vessels—before they enter the skull, and very rarely it is possible to treat this with surgery. Another, treatable cause of impaired blood supply to the brain is when little clots or emboli are thrown off from the left auricle of the heart and enter the cerebral circulation. This is associated with fibrillation of the auricle (a feature of heart disease, due to old rheumatic fever, an overactive thyroid gland, high blood pressure or a poor blood supply to the wall of the heart itself). The consequent inefficient contraction of the auricle allows clot to form within a pouch which opens off the main cavity, and from time to time small pieces of this clot break off and enter the brain. The treatment is by an anticoagulant drug to reduce the blood's tendency to clot, and digitalis or digoxin to help the heart contract more efficiently. By these means I remember restoring to complete mental normality a grossly confused lady known to have heart disease who had become too disturbed to be treated in a general medical ward. Heart failure can cause confusion by reducing the cardiac output. Sudden heart failure may be due to coronary thrombosis, of which confusion rather than chest pain can be the presenting sign. Inflammation of the temporal artery (arteritis) is an occasional cause of subacute confusion.

b. Poor *oxygenation* of the blood in the lungs, because of bronchitis emphysema, asthma or pneumonia (which, causing part of the lung to solidify and thus not be available for the exchange of gases, produces confusion by hypoxia as well as infection).

c. 'Poor *blood*' i.e. blood which is anaemic, or low in haemoglobin (the pigment attached to which oxygen is carried from the lungs to the brain). Anaemia may result from a lack of iron or folic acid in the diet, from chronic bleeding (e.g. from a peptic ulcer, a cancer or piles) or from the inability of the body to manufacture vitamin B_{12}—pernicious anaemia. (Lack of B_{12} effects the brain directly, as well as through the anaemia.)

Anaemia is rarely the direct cause of an acute confusional state, though it may well contribute to one, but may be responsible for the subacute state, and can even mimic dementia.

3. *Malnutrition*, where the diet is deficient in vitamins of the B group—chiefly thiamine, riboflavin and nicotinic acid. This may result from a generally deficient diet due to poverty, helplessness or depression, from eccentricity and food-fads, or from alcoholism, which is by no means unknown in the elderly. The combination of vitamin B deficiency with alcoholic intoxication is responsible for delirium tremens.

4. *Dehydration*, from inadequate intake of water, usually due to extreme infirmity or deep depression. Dehydration is associated with electrolyte imbalance, which causes more confusion, following prolonged diarrhoea and/or vomiting.

5. *Metabolic disorder*, such as failure of the kidneys (producing uraemia) and of the liver, e.g. associated with cirrhosis.

6. *Endocrine disorder*, the most important being *diabetes*. Uncontrolled diabetes can cause a very dangerous state of ketosis, which may well produce transitory confusion before going on to coma.

Probably a more common cause of confusion in diabetes, though, is irregular and injudicious self-administration of the very drugs given to regulate the disorder which, taken in excess, lower the blood sugar below the normal level.

Both over- and underactivity of the *thyroid* gland can cause confusion of the subacute kind. Thyrotoxicosis (thyroid overactivity) is more likely to produce a typically delirious picture, whereas in hypothyroidism the confusion is more chronic, mimicking dementia, and associated with lethargy and depression or paranoia.

7. *Trauma*, e.g. following a fracture, head injury or surgery. A fracture is not easily overlooked as a cause of confusion, though I have known inability to walk on a broken thigh to be ascribed to hysteria. Confusional states can complicate all surgical operations, particularly major ones and those on the eyes and the heart; doubtless the anaesthetic is sometimes as much responsible as the surgery. One consequence of head injury must be carefully excluded whenever there is fluctuating confusion over the course of several weeks, accompanied by varying neurological signs: the chronic subdural haematoma. This is a clot, formed as a result of bleeding beneath the outer covering of the brain following a blow to the head which may have seemed at the time quite trifling. The effects are those of rapidly progressive cerebral tumour, and may prove fatal unless the correct diagnosis is made and the clot evacuated. However, the more usual after-effects of head injury of any severity is concussion which can be followed by confusion lasting for several weeks.

8. *Intracranial disorder*, e.g. cerebral tumour which might be primary but in the elderly is much more likely to be secondary to cancer elsewhere in the body, such as the lung; and cerebral abscess, sometimes due to ear infection. Infections directly affecting the brain—meningitis and encephalitis—are rare in this age group. Epilepsy arising from the temporal lobe of the brain can produce a 'twilight state' which is a form of delirium, but this is very unlikely to occur for the first time in old age.

9. *Intoxication by chemical agents*. Alas, this is mainly iatrogenic which means 'caused by the doctor'. All drugs are potential poisons, especially to the elderly who break them down and eliminate more slowly than younger patients. Ironically, the very drugs used to control confusion may add to it. Tranquillisers can do more harm than good, for example by causing drowsiness or dropping the blood pressure. Even supposedly safe sleeping tablets like Nitrazepam (Mogadon) can cause a hangover of reduced alertness next morning. and if the drug is given nightly the effect may

be cumulative. It is not difficult to give an excess of digoxin, the drug chiefly used in the treatment of heart disease, and where a diuretic is also given (to relieve the body of the fluid which accumulates in heart failure) there is the danger of excreting too much potassium and producing a state of confusion and langour. Steroids are powerful drugs, used in the treatment of asthma, rheumatoid arthritis and some other forms of inflammation, which have serious side-effects, some of which are mental—depression, exaltation, paranoia and confusion. A lady of 80 was terrorising a medical ward, despite her advanced years, by her bemused belligerence; she had been put on a large dose of prednisone for very severe asthma, and was exhibiting a 'steroid psychosis'. The problem in treatment was to reduce the drug to a level which did not effect her mind while continuing to relieve the asthma. L-dopa, which has proved a great boon to some sufferers from Parkinsonism, can also cause a state of rather fatuous, euphoric confusion, and again there is great difficulty in adjusting the dosage to do physical good without mental harm. Benzhexol (Artane), another drug more commonly used for Parkinsonism, can also produce confusion (and paranoia). Benzhexol is an anticholinergic drug. Most antidepressants are also anticholinergic, and they too may occasionally cause acute confusion. Drugs which lower blood pressure and blood sugar also sometimes cause confusion. Drugs are two-edged weapons, and must be used with especial caution in the elderly who not only metabolise them relatively slowly but also, being forgetful, take them unreliably.

10. *Hypothermia* has already been mentioned (Ch. 2) as a hazard to old people in very cold weather, and this causes drowsiness and confusion, followed by coma.

11. Severe *pain*, such as that caused by herpes (shingles), acute glaucoma (sudden increase in the pressure within the eyeball) or even toothache; and chronic discomfort, notably that of faecal impaction (constipation so severe that the faeces must be removed by hand) and itching sometimes cause confusion.

12. Finally, although delirium is usually an expression of physical disorder, *psychological stress* of catastrophic intensity, such as a sudden bereavement or a move either expected or wanted, sometimes precipitates acute confusion.

The most important disorder from which delirium needs to be distinguished is *dementia*, of which the chief characteristic is also confusion. The distinction matters, because dementia is an untreatable disease, requiring long-term management, whereas delirium, once diagnosed, nearly always responds to treatment if it is given soon enough. Clouding of consciousness, fluctuations in confusion, illusions and hallucinations are not typical of dementia, and the presence of signs of a physical illness sufficient to produce the confusion indicates delirium; however, where the patient is very disturbed these signs may not be readily elicited. For and away the most useful differentiation is by means of the history. If the confusion has developed within the past few days, or even weeks, then it must be due to delirium, the cause of which should be energetically sought. Dementia never presents with such a short history. It is, of course, quite possible for delirium to occur in someone who is already demented, so even if confusion has been present for a long time the history must establish whether, and in what way, it has worsened recently. Obviously the patient will not be able to give a proper account of himself, so the story must be obtained from someone who knows him. It is not just the doctor's job to get this information, but the duty of any member of the staff team who is present when an informant is available.

Acute *mania* in the elderly may closely resemble delirium in the early stages. The presence of a family or previous history of attacks of mania or depression, and the absence of physical illness will suggest the diagnosis, and after a few days the confusion usually subsides, and manic features come to the fore.

Coolness and commonsense are needed to make the right diagnosis in the face of very disturbed behaviour, while premature sedation or hasty disposal to a mental hospital can do harm.

Assessment of the physical condition requires at the very least a full physical examination (and to claim that the patient is 'too disturbed to examine' is no more acceptable than failing to wash out the stomach of an attempted suicide on the grounds that the patient will not co-operate) including a rectal examination, urine testing, a record of the temperature (not neglecting the low-reading thermometer in case of hypothermia) pulse and rate of respiration, X-rays of the chest and skull, and the blood picture. More specialised investigations will be suggested by the original findings. The electroencephalogram will show a decrease in frequency related to clouding of consciousness, and is not otherwise informative unless there is a localised brain lesion.

After diagnosis comes *treatment*, and the first decision to be made is where the patient is to be treated. If he is not too ill or disturbed, if the home is habitable and if there are people there to look after him, then the familiar surroundings of home will suit him best. The doctor will call daily, the District Nurse more often, if necessary, to prescribe and administer the appropriate treatment and watch progress.

If hospital is required, though, it should be a general and not a mental hospital. The latter lacks facilities to assess and treat serious physical illness, to which disturbed behaviour is of secondary importance. Perhaps the ideal placement for the acutely confused old person is a psychogeriatric assessment unit—a medical ward in a general hospital jointly staffed by psychiatrist and geriatrician, and nurses with a psychiatric as well as a general training (see Ch. 12).

Apart from specific treatment for the underlying disease, the patient needs nourishment and rest. Skilled, patient management is required to see that he gets these. An adequate fluid intake is essential; not less than 2 litres/day. If this is not taken by mouth, it must be given intravenously as 5 per cent glucose; however, care must be then observed in case the patient is precipitated into heart failure. An appetising balanced diet is desirable, but essential nutrients can be given to the very feeble in the form of the semi-fluid Complan. A course of the B group and other vitamins is normally given as well, by intramuscular or intravenous injections—Parentrovite, one pair of ampoules daily for a week.

A watch must be kept on the output of urine and the opening of the bowels. One litre of urine should be passed every 24 hours, and a quantity of much less than this indicates either dehydration, requiring a greater intake of fluid, or retention. Urinary retention and constipation are uncomfortable conditions likely to aggravate confusion and distress, and must be relieved, with the aid of a catheter and an enema if necessary.

Bright, plain well-lit surroundings, the presence of a familiar object or two (such as a clock or a well-loved photograph) quiet, physical comfort and an unchanging routine all reduce alarm and promote rest without recourse to sedatives. If the staff are composed, confident and caring, constantly reassuring and re-orientating the patient, recovery is likely to be smooth and rapid. On the other hand, if they are frightened and rejecting, knocking the patient flat with drugs, pushing him out of sight in a side room and neglecting even his basic physical needs for nutrition and warmth, they may kill him. I am sorry to say that I have had on occasion literally to rescue a patient from such a situation by transfering him to a more accepting environment.

Sedation needs to be used sparingly, but has a place where the patient is so restless that he is getting exhausted. Tranquillisers are useful: the longest established is chlorpromazine (Largactil), by mouth or injection, the only serious disadvantage of which is that it may drop the blood pressure somewhat alarmingly. Thioridazine (Melleril) is a milder tranquilliser of the same kind but without any such tendency. Particularly useful because it calms without putting the patient to sleep is haloperidol (Seranace), by mouth or injection. This has the snag that it readily causes shaking, stiffness, muscular spasms and drooling, but these side-effects can usually be counteracted by one of the drugs given for Parkinsonism, say orphenadrine (Disipal), or procyclidine (Kemadrine) by injection, through the same needle by which the tranquilliser has just been given. Chlormethiazole (Heminevrin) is another useful sedative for the delirious. If it is also necessary to give sleeping tablets at night, a benzodiazepine like nitrozepam (Mogadon) is commonly provided, though triazolam (Halcion) and temazepam (Normison, Euhypnos) might sometimes be preferred for their shorter length of action. Chloral hydrate is a tried and true sleeping draught which some old people take more readily than tablets; a tablet form of the same drug is dichloralphenazone (Welldorm). Barbiturates, which can themselves be a cause of confusion, and paraldehyde are now obsolete (for doses of these drugs see Ch.14).

REFERENCES

Lipowski Z J 1980 Delirium updated. Comprehensive Psychiatry 21: 190

6

Dementia

If not the most common, dementia is surely the most serious psychiatric disorder of old age. Ten per cent of those over 65 years of age are demented, and in half of these the condition is at least moderately severe. Yet only one-fifth of the demented elderly are cared for in any kind of institution.

The essential features of dementia, the picture produced by chronic and extensive (global) brain disease, are intellectual deterioration, an impaired memory especially for recent events and disorientation, all occurring without any drowsiness (clouding of consciousness) and persisting. Most definitions of dementia emphasize its insidious onset, chronic and progressive course and irreversibility. While this is generally correct, there are occasional exceptions where the decline appears to halt or there may actually be a modest clinical improvement. In any case, a definition so closely committed to the course of the disorder is unsatisfactory for early cases, where that course has yet to be determined. I therefore prefer Lipowski's (1980) definition, 'a global cognitive disorder that is relatively stable and unaccompanied by fluctuating disturbance of wakefulness and attention and has lasted more than three months' or Marsden's (1978) succinct 'The syndrome of a global disturbance of higher mental functions in an alert patient'.

Dementia can be a devastating disease eroding personality as well as intellect and damaging relationships irreparably. Sometimes it seems as if the true self dies long before the body's death, and in the intervening years a smudged caricature disintegrates noisily and without dignity into chaos. Until recently the challenge presented by this tragic disorder has been largely ignored. The close identification of dementia with irreversible ageing has meant that clinicians and research scientists have turned their backs, looking for more rewarding scope for their skills. Having made the dreadful discovery of 'cerebral atrophy' neurologists have lost interest, while physicians and surgeons resent the 'blocking' of an acute bed when dementia delays discharge. Residential homes tended to shun the confused elderly, and the burden of care has been left to families, general practitioners and social services in the community, and to the back wards of geriatric and psychiatric hospitals. Here, far removed from the centres of excellence, like the teaching hospitals, where diverse experts meet and can fruitfully discuss complex problems to which no single specialty can have the answer (and dementia is, par excellence, one such) barely basic care is given, while detailed observations, investigations and appraisal to understand the course of the condition and how it may be influenced is very scant.

Recogition, owever, that with the inexorable ageing of the population, and especially the increase in those over 65, who are most at risk, dementia threatens to overwhelm the health and social services, led Britain's Department of Health and Social Services in 1972 to issue *Services for Mental Illness Related to Old age*, with clear guidance about where the demented should be looked after, by whom and the scale of provision to be made for them. In 1977, after a conference including neurologists, neuropathologists, neurobiochemists, geneticists, an immunologist, psychiatrists and geriatricians the Medical Research Council publicised its interest in dementia research to the scientific community. Very soon afterwards the discovery that there is a specific neurotransmitter defect in the most serious dementia of old age, Alzheimer's disease (see later) sharpened this interest by shifting its focus from the dead or dying nerve cell to a potentially remediable biochemical abnormality. In the United States rehabilitative techniques to improve the memory of the demented were developed by Folsom (1967) and have now been enthusiastically adopted elsewhere. The growth of the subspecialty of psychogeriatrics, particularly in Britain, has meant that now many more psychiatrists are actively interested in the condition. The development of computerised axial tomography (CAT) is enabling wonderfully clear pictures to be taken of the brain which could previously only be obtained (and then in an inferior form) by the potentially dangerous injection of dyes and air. Ever less gradually dementia is getting the attention it demands.

The main forms of dementia in old age are *Alzheimer's disease* (senile dementia) and *multi infarct* (or atherosclerotic) dementia. There is probably a third, more benign form, which is closely related to ageing.

ALZHEIMER'S DISEASE (Senile dementia)

This, the worst form of dementia, appears to predominate in

women, and as women more and more outnumber men the older
they get, it is unfortunately also the most common. It pursues,
usually, an unremitting course over a couple or several years, from
impairment of the higher mental abilities, such as judgement, self
criticism and abstract thinking in the early stages to virtual disin-
tegration of the intellect and personality and an ultimate state of
incoherent incontinence. *Forgetfulness* is an early sign and rapidly
becomes extensive and disabling. The oldest memories tend to be
the last to go (Ribot's law) and hence the characteristic dwelling in
the past: many dementing old wives or widows when asked who
they are will give their maiden names, forgetting all about the forty
odd years of their marriage! This *dysmnesia* is usually soon accompanied and complicated by *dysphasia* (difficulty in finding the right
words, or understanding what is said) which impedes speech and
comprehension. Typical, too, of Alzheimer's disease is *dyspraxia*, a
difficulty in putting movements together due to malfunction of the
parietal lobe of the brain, which is a severe handicap in, say, dressing and feeding. Gross neurological signs, however, such as spasticity or paralysis, are rare and late. Interest rapidly dwindles, and
is replaced by vacant *apathy*. *Emotions* may become *labile*, tears,
laughter and anger being easily provoked, and as readily subsiding.
Usually there is little or no *insight* into what is happening, the patient blandly disclaiming the defects in her memory and her capacity to care for herself which are so evident to others. Sometimes
self-awareness is kept away by the mental mechanisms of *denial*—
'there's nothing wrong with my memory' (the memory gaps may
be filled by *confabulation*, or making up stories) and *projection*—
'the reason I can't find my things is because everybody keeps
taking them'. Thus there can be a very troublesome *paranoid phase*
during which the family and friends can be very hurt by vigorous,
if irrational accusations; eventually, though, with the continuing
progress of the dementia, the patient is no longer able to form her
delusions. *Habits deteriorate* partly because of apathy and not
caring, partly because propriety and social behaviour are lost, and
partly because of dyspraxia. Food is slopped, dress is careless and
slovenly, washing perfunctory and reluctant and control over the
bladder (less often of the bowel) erratic. *Incontinence* and unex-
plained *aggression* are very hard for households to tolerate, though
very rarely indeed is a demented patient's hostility in the least
dangerous. *Wandering* can be a great problem; sometimes the patient insists that the home in which she has lived for the last 30
years is not hers, and that her husband is a stranger, and she goes
off in search of her mother. She may knock up her neighbours in

the middle of the night, causing great annoyance, or, more seriously, gets lost. Leaving the gas on unlit and interference with electrical appliances, are, understandably, other causes of great anxiety.

The demented old person living alone is in obvious danger of self neglect. If she is with her spouse or children, the problem is more theirs—how they are to manage her and cope with their own mixed feelings. If admitted because of dementia to hospital or an old people's home, the patient is likely to survive two years or so; the more helpless she appears on admission. the less likely she is to live long. It used to be thought that the natural end of dementia was to be bedridden, with contracted limbs and bedsores. We now know that this was the effect of putting the patient to bed, and since the policy has been to keep her up and about death is more often due to a bout of pneumonia, a heart attack or (the inevitable and entirely acceptable occasional consequence of encouraging activity) a fractured femur.

Alzheimer's disease is a disease and by no means simply due to ageing, though dementia (like heart and respiratory disease) becomes a greater hazard with advancing years. It is fairly rare before the age of 65, though the disease originally described by Alzheimer (1907) occurred in much younger patients, and was thought to be a separate disorder with a stronger family history; however, the abnormalities in the brains of older and younger victims are identical. Kay and colleagues (1970) showed that dementia exists in two to three per cent of those aged between 65 and 74, in twice as many of those 75 to 79, and in no less than 22 per cent of those over 80. The age relationship is striking, but the corollary is that almost 80 per cent of octogenarians and older are not suffering from dementia.

The cause of Alzheimer's disease is at present quite unknown, though there are several theories. It has long been assumed that the dementia is the consequence of an acceleration in the death of nerve cells or neurones so that too few survive for thoughts, memories, intentions and reactions to be mediated normally. The loss of grey matter in the demented brain, with shrinking and smoothing of the surface or cortex, the loss of clefts or grooves or gyri and enlargement of the ventricles and a lower brain weight than is normal at that age certainly suggest, but do not prove that there is a loss of neurones, which are exceedingly difficult to count. At a colloquium on the subject of Alzheimer's disease in Edinburgh in 1979 the eminent neuropathologist Wiesniwski observed that 'the neurone is sick, but not beyond recovery'.

The characteristic abnormalities in the brains of sufferers from

Alzheimer's disease, visible only with a microscope, are *neurofibrillary tangles* and *senile plaques*. The former are due to changes in the tubular fibres or nerve processes radiating from the nerve cell to connect at the synapses with the processes of other nerve cells. The electron microscope has shown that the normally straight neurotubules are replaced by a pair of filaments coiled round each other (PHF—paired helical filaments) which give the tangled appearance. The likely cause of this is an alteration in the protein of the neurotubule. Plaques are infiltrations of amyloid, a waxy starchy substance which fills the space between the capillaries or tiny blood vessels to the brain. Plaques could be collections of degenerated nerve fibres, damaged by the process described above, or a response to some toxin derived from the blood.

Plaques can be induced in the brains of mice by strains of the organism which causes scrapie in sheep. This provides a handy animal model of dementia for experimental purposes and the faint possibility of a connection between Alzheimer's disease and a rare group of neurological disorders which may be spread by an infective agent, known as the transmissible spongy encephalopathies. These include *kuru,* which is confined to New Guinea and allegedly acquired by cannibals who eat the infected brains of their victims, and an extremely obscure pre-senile dementia called Jakob Creutzfeld disease. This has been transmitted to rhesus monkeys experimentally, and rarely by corneal transplants from diseased donors and electrodes touching the brain for a special EEG. The theory that Alzheimer's disease is congenital, transmitted by a 'slow' virus which takes almost a life time to show its effects, has been advanced, but at present seems decidedly far-fetched.

Of more practical value, perhaps, is the already mentioned discovery of a neurotransmitter deficiency in the limbic system (that part of the brain especially concerned with memory) of patients dying with Alzheimer's disease. Neurotransmitters transfer information across the gap (synapses) between the ends of nerve processes linking the nerve cells. The substance depleted in Alzheimer's disease (compared with old people dying without that disorder) is acetyl choline, and the neurones which use that transmitter seem especially vulnerable to whatever causes the dementia (Davies & Maloney, 1976; Perry et al, 1977). Whether this is an intrinsic part of the process of dementia and relevant to its clinical manifestations is as yet unknown. However, deficiency of another neurotransmitter, dopamine, is relevant to the crippling Parkinson's disease, and at least partially remediable by giving L dopa, which raises the level of dopamine at the nerve endings, and there is a similar hope (as yet unrealised) that a substance may be found which will firstly raise the level of acetyl choline at the relevant synapses and secondly thus improve mental functioning in dementia.

There is certainly an hereditary factor in senile dementia, for if one of a pair of non-identical twins develops the condition, the risk of the other twin getting it is 8 per cent; whereas if the twins are identical, which means that genetically they are exactly the same, the risk increases to 43 per cent (Kallman, 1951). Also, a Scandinavian study has shown that one's risk of suffering senile dementia is four times as great as that of the general population if one has close relative with the disorder (Larsson, Sjogren & Jacobson,1963). There is a connection between Down's syndrome (Mongolism) and Alzheimer's disease. Almost all mongols over 35 show the characteristic changes in their brains (Olsen & Shaw, 1969).

It has been suggested that senile dementia particularly afflicts the lower classes and those with an already abnormal personality. However, it is unlikely that the condition is any respector of persons, though it is very probable that the difficult and underprivileged will be more readily admitted to mental hospital.

It has also been alleged that the changes found in the brain post mortem are often inconsistent with the degree of dementia shown during life, and the suggestion has been made that it is not so much the degree of brain damage, but the personality's reaction to it which determines the severity of dementia. However, elegant work by Corsellis (1962) in London and Blessed, Tomlinson & Roth (1968) at Newcastle-upon-Tyne has shown quite a close relationship between the severity of dementia in life (for example, as recorded on a rating scale) and pathological changes (chiefly the quantity of neurofibrillary tangles and senile plaques) in the brain after death.

MULTI-INFARCT (ATHERSCLEROTIC) DEMENTIA

This results from the throttling of the arteries supplying the brain (as described on p. 32) by atheroma. The course is typically be a series of 'little strokes'—episodes of confusion sometimes associated with minor neurological signs (slurring of speech, weakness down one side of the body, or in a single limb) due to sudden inadequacy of the cerebral circulation, either because a vessel has become completely blocked, or because for some reason the blood pressure has dropped below the level necessary to force the blood through some of the narrowed arteries. The network of arteries to the brain is very rich, and after a few days or weeks the circulation is restored. There is then clinical improvement, or even full recovery, until the next episode, which takes place in a matter of weeks, months or sometimes not for more than a year. Eventually, however, after a succession of such bouts there is less and less recovery, until by a process of 'step-ladder' deterioration dementia as profound as the senile variety develops.

Other signs of brain damage than dementia indicate the atherosclerotic process. Complaints of dizziness are quite common in the early stages, actual 'blackouts' are not uncommon, and later there may even be fits. High blood pressure is present in about half the cases. Slurring of speech, Parkinsonism (stiffness and shakiness of the voluntary muscles) weakness of one side of the face and/or body, defects of the visual field (inability to see things to one or other side) and spasticity of the limbs are common neurological signs. Typically the atherosclerotic has a shuffling gait, with little steps—the 'marche à petit pas'. There are frequently, also, signs of heart disease and of atherosclerosis in other blood vessels in the body than those supplying the brain.

Nevertheless, it is often surprising that, on the one hand, a man can suffer severe atherosclerotic dementia with only minor physical disability, while on the other a patient with a serious stroke may show no intellectual impairment. The explanation is probably that in dementia the blockage mainly effects the smaller vessels, nearer the brain's surface, and thus mainly spares the tracts lying deeper in the brain which govern movement, whereas major strokes result from obstruction of a major vessel while the other arteries may be relatively free from disease.

Although the disease is widespread in the brain, the cortex is less uniformly affected than in senile dementia, and the patchiness of the lesions, together with the tendency towards some return of function after an incident of occlusion, makes for fluctuations, inconsistency and an intriguing variety of clinical pictures.

Confusion is inconstant; an old man may be muddled in the morning, lucid and alert in the afternoon, rambling and disorientated again in the evening. (It is therefore important, if one is required to assess such a patient, not to rely exclusively on how he performs at a single interview but to pay close attention to the history, otherwise one may have unfair suspicions that he is being wilfully misrepresented.)

Emotionalism is sometimes very marked. Weeping may be induced so easily as to suggest the Mock Turtle in *Alice in Wonderland*. However, the distress is not always shallow. The personality is relatively well preserved until a late stage in the dementia, and the consequent insight into the failing memory can cause profound depression and even suicide. Apparently, though, this depression is not wholly reactive to the dementia, for there is a family history of depressive illness in atherosclerotic depressives even more often than in elderly sufferers from depressive illness alone (Post, 1962). There may be a constitutional link between atherosclerosis and depression; anyway, the dementia can precipitate true depressive illness in the predisposed.

A paranoid phase is as common as in senile dementia. At this stage a common reaction to questions designed to test the memory is one of extreme indignation—the 'catastrophic' response—often leading to abrupt termination of the interview, without, of course, the intellectual deficit being exposed. Paranoid delusions in dementia are always directed against those at hand, and never achieve the elaborate consistent quality of those which characterise paraphrenia.

Though relatively well preserved, the personality is not undamaged. Impairment of judgement and self-criticism sometimes precede memory failure. A lady with a history of high blood pressure, a recent confusional episode (and depression) was very anxious about her appointment to see me, fearing that I would have her 'put away'. There was no question of this, and in fact at interview she gave a pretty good account of herself, and though she went into unnecessary detail and said some things two or three times over, her orientation was entirely correct. However, towards the end of our conversation she handed over a great many pieces of paper, on which she had that morning recorded her understanding of a television programme she had been watching. This was to prove her sanity (which was not really in doubt) but instead it demonstrated her defective judgement, in attempting the proof so laboriously. Deterioration of these higher abilities matters most in those who have to exercise considerable skill from positions of major responsibility, e.g. judges, surgeons, and of course, politicians.

Sometimes the usual pattern is reversed, and personality degenerates while the memory is relatively unimpaired. Presumably in such cases the frontal lobes of the brain, which seem to have much to do with the finer features of personality such as unselfishness, the moral sense and restraint, are affected earlier by the atherosclerosis. A common complaint by the spouse is that the patient was never easy to live with but recently has become impossible—completely self-centred, callous, cruel, coarse, crude and explosively irritable; yet performance of intellectual tests is within normal limits for the age. One such patient was repeatedly admitted to a mental hospital on a short-term compulsory order at weekends (usually when neither the doctor sending nor the doctor receiving him knew him beforehand), following a domestic crisis. As he was unwilling to stay, however, and as there seemed inadequate grounds for his detention under the Mental Health Act he was allowed to take his discharge later in the week. Back and forth this hapless wanderer went between his home and hospital, until one day he disappeared. Months later his body was found in a copse just within the hospital gates. Autopsy was able to demonstrate that ironically he had died of a massive brain haemorrhage while taking himself off home.

The final picture of multi-infarct dementia is that of any advanced dementia, with severe loss of memory and dysphasia, dyspraxia to the point of helplessness and incontinence. Physically infirmity is more marked than at the comparable stage of senile dementia, and death, quite often from a serious stroke, is not long delayed.

Post mortem the brain may present a 'moth-eaten' appearance, the surface being marked by many infarcts (soft, discoloured areas of tissue which died before the patient because of an insufficient blood supply); on the other hand it may seem quite normal to the naked eye, and the effects of the disease are only detectable under the microscope.

Table 1 Comparison between Alzheimer's disease, multi-infarct dementia and benign senescent forgetfulness

	Alzheimer's	Multi-infarct	Benign
Age of onset	45 onwards	45 onwards	After 80
Sex	Commoner in women	Commonest in men	Commoner in women
Course	Progressive & global	'Step ladder' and focal	Slow, mainly affecting memory
Dysphasia & dyspraxia	Soon	Sooner or later	Absent
Impairment of insight, intellect and personality	Early	Late	Late
Physical symptoms	Absent	Present (headache, dizziness)	Absent
Physical signs	Few and late (e.g. grasp reflex)	Frequent (tremors, paralysis, spasticity)	Absent

Both Alzheimer's disease and multi-infarct dementia are fairly common in the elderly, and it is not surprising that the brains of about 20 per cent of demented patients should show signs of both disease processes. However, the distinction between the two is worth making clinically, if possible, because the short-term future and thus the plan of management for each are different. Alzheimer's disease is likely simply to get worse, while there may be a measure of recovery, if only temporary, from the effects of a recent infarct. The essential differences are listed in table 1, together with those features which may distinguish a benign form of dementia.

A BENIGN DEMENTIA

As has been mentioned in Chapter Two, Kral (1965) postulated a distinction between dementia and 'benign senescent forgetfulness'. Whereas in the former there is total forgetting of events, in the latter they are half, imperfectly remembered. Also there is a tendency to remember the essentials for day to day living, even though general knowledge and awareness of current events is poor. Although Roth & Myers (1969) found that the condition is much less benign and more typical of dementia after a year, there is circumstantial evidence that there may be a less severe dementia swelling the numbers of those so afflicted at an advanced age.

McDonald (1968) noted that there were two groups of patients admitted to Kew Hospital (Melbourne) with senile dementia. One suffered dysphasia and dyspraxia as well as forgetfulness, the other memory impairment alone. The latter, although significantly older, survived significantly longer. Then Hare (1978) noted a very similar difference in the prospects for patients admitted to a psychogeriatric assessment ward. Nearly half of those who were dyspraxic and dysphasic as well as confused died within six months and of 56, only three were out of hospital, while those who were simply forgetful nearly all survived and were discharged (p. 48). Finally Jacoby (1980) reporting on the use of the CAT scan in demented subjects said that atrophy of the cortex and enlargement of the ventricles were less apparent in the oldest than in those who were not quite so old.

This suggests that there is a group of very old people whose dementia comprises forgetfulness alone. Hard though it may be to teach very old dogs new tricks (or even old ones!) these may be especiallly suitable for reality orientation therapy, and thus the effects of the alarming increase in the numbers of the demented among the very old may possibly to some degree be mitigated.

Other causes of dementia in old age are rare, but sometimes treatable. They include syphilis, which may not show signs of having affected the brain until 20 years after the original infection. General paralysis of the insane, the picturesque term given to neurosyphilitic dementia, used to account for one in 20 admissions to mental hospitals at the turn of the century, but is now rare, despite increasing promiscuity, because syphilis can be cured at all stages by large doses of penicillin. Nevertheless, the diagnosis must often be considered, however infrequently it is confirmed by blood tests. Cerebral tumour is another condition which can cause dementia before the physical effects are apparent, and may be treatable if benign (i.e. simply causing local pressure) rather than malignant (invasive). Cerebral tumour must be considered where ever there are neurological signs, or when investigations suggest an abnormality on one side of the brain only.

A condition known as *normal pressure (communicating) hydrocephalus* should be considered where confusion, incontinence and unsteadiness of gait (ataxia) are associated with a past history of head injury or brain (subarachnoid) haemorrhage, or meningitis. It is suggested by gross ventricular enlargement on the CAT scan, but studies of the flow of the cerebrospinal fluid which bathes the brain and fills the ventricles are needed to confirm the diagnosis. It may be remediable by a shunt operation which returns excess cerebrospinal fluid to the right atrium of the heart by way of the jugular vein.

It is suggested by Albert (1979) that there may be a *subcortical* form of dementia in which the lesion or defect is in the mid brain. The very rare Steele Richardson syndrome is an instance. Here Parkinsonian rigidity of the trunk and certain abnormal eye movements are associated with a mental slowing rather like dementia, and it is suggested that mental impairment following the onset of Parkinson's disease may sometimes be due to a subcortical deficit, possibly of a biochemial nature within the recticular system which activates the cortex, and therefore possibly amenable to some kind of substitution therapy. The nature of any subcortical dementia, however, and its reversibility are still largely matters for speculation.

Dementia must be distinguished from acute and subacute confusional states, chiefly by the history, as explained in the previous chapter (pp. 35–36). Dementia is a damning diagnosis in that it virtually rules out the possibility of treatment, and should therefore never be made in haste or lightly. In particular such causes of a prolonged subacute confusional state as hypothyroidism, deficiency of vitamin B12 and chronic subdural haematoma must be carefully excluded.

Attention has been drawn above to the frequent association of multi-infarct dementia with depression.

However, not every confused elderly depressed patient is demented (or delirious). Sometimes when old people develop severe depressive illness they appear genuinely confused also, but the confusion is wholly secondary to the depression, and clears when the depression lifts. The distinction between true and this depressive *pseudodementia* is not always easy. A previous or family history of depression, the onset of depressive symptoms before memory impairment, the presence of malaise, agitation, and peevishness if not frank melancholy and despair, early waking, a tendency to be worst at the beginning of the day and the patient's failure in any way to deny his confusion or to confabulate, all suggest a depressive basis, but a 'therapeutic trial' of antidepressive drugs or even electroplexy may be necessary to confirm the diagnosis.

A man of 70 who had waited on his demanding, asthmatic wife hand and foot since his retirement became unable—or unwilling—to do so any more, and she complained bitterly. He was withdrawn, restless and odd. He ignored many questions, and his few answers were brief, vague and long-delayed. He would not relax, and he interfered with his wife's attempts to do housework and cooking, as he did not want her to use any electricity. In hospital he was suspected to have cancer of the lung. He was a cigarette smoker, had lost a lot of weight recently, and there were sinister shadows on his chest X-rays. He refused a bronchoscopy, which might have confirmed that diagnosis, and because of his strangeness, vagueness and rather negative, uncooperative attitude it was thought that he might be demented. However, the geriatrician who saw him found no serious confusion, was impressed by the lack of incontinence, and was unwilling to apply the dementia label. The patient was sent home and a few months later I was asked to see him. Physically he was no worse, which made cancer unlikely. I found him untidy, but not dirty, evasive, though not hostile, uneasy, but not actually depressed, and uninformative but not greatly disorientated. Tests by a clinical psychologist showed decided impairment of his ability to learn, or to tackle puzzles and problems, in comparison with his knowledge of words, which was at the level of good average intelligence. This discrepancy between old knowledge and present intellectual performance is typical of dementia. Nevertheless, the fact that he was mentally little worse than a year previously was inconsistent with dementia, and his withdrawal, agitation and miserliness (in respect of the electricity) were consistent with depression, though he had never previously suffered from such disorder. It was

considered that the likely diagnosis was either cerebral atherosclerosis, which had not yet reached the stage of clinical dementia, or
depressive pseudodementia. He was given a course of six electrical
treatments, it being thought that he had something to gain and little to lose, and he made a dramatic improvement. He became
cheerful, active, alert, sociable, helpful—in fact, his old self. The
psychological tests were repeated, and now showed a return to normal intellectual function; the discrepancy between 'old' and 'new'
knowledge had been abolished.

To establish the *diagnosis* of dementia as full a history as possible must be obtained from the patient and those who know him.
Ideally the assessment should be made in the first instance at home,
where the relevant social circumstances, the practical problems and
the possible resources can be best appreciated. A full physical examination follows, and routine investigations include serology (to
exclude syphilis), skull X-ray, as well as tests of the blood (blood
picture and biochemical profile) and urine and chest X-ray. Elec-
tro-encephalography, brain scan and CAT scan are generally reserved for those under 75 in whom the history and physical examination strongly suggest a cerebral tumour, abscess, haematoma or hydrocephalus. Otherwise, although they are of academic interest, the cost of these investigations is not really justified by the
benefits they may confer.

The EEG gives little reliable information where dementia is early
or doubtful, and though there are often gross abnormalities when
the condition is well advanced, the diagnosis is then hardly in
doubt. However, when the recording shows an abnormality confined to one side or area of the brain, particularly slow, irregular
waves, a tumour, abscess or haematoma is a distinct possibility and
further investigation is needed. Tumours, infarcts and cortical atrophy show up well on the CAT scan, (though ten per cent of old
people who show atrophy appear mentally normal!) and gross enlargement of the ventricles might suggest communicating hydrocephalus. Lumbar puncture (the tapping of cerebrospinal fluid
through a needle inserted in the base of the spine) is only necessary
if infection of the brain or bleeding beneath one of its coverings is
suspected; in the presence of a tumour it can be dangerous.

Psychological testing is of limited help in diagnosis. Where the
psychiatrist is unsure about the presence of dementia, the results of
psychological testing are often equivocal, and the uncertainty remains. Where the diagnosis seems pretty likely on clinical grounds,
the patient is often too unattentive, distractible, erratic or otherwise uncooperative to be tested. No tests wholly distinguish brain

damaged subjects from those whose performance may be impaired by depressive perturbation and preoccupation (see the case history above) or other distracting functional mental disorder. Patients with pseudodementia may be just as unable as the truly demented to remember an address, a number or a story which they have just been told, or to do simple mental arithmetic, though they are more likely to remember the correct dates of important events in their own lives, to know of significant world occurrances and to be correctly orientated.

Tests are needed which are reliable, valid (i.e. measure what they are supposed to measure) sensitive (so that small and subtle changes may be discerned), acceptable to subjects and repeatable without distortion of the scores by practice effect. Though none now in use match up to all these requirements, the following are among those sometimes helpful in the assessment of elderly patients.

The Wechsler Adult Intelligence Scale (WAIS) indicates how the old person's score compares with those of a sample of normal people of like age. The scale comprises tests of vocabulary (which give a good idea of the previous level of intelligence) and of performance which indicates present ability. Performance signficantly worse than vocabulary suggests dementia (but see case history above).

The Walton Black Modified Word Learning Test aims to teach subjects the meanings of ten words they have been found not to know, and is scored by the number of times they have to be told before they get six out of the ten words right. This tends to distinguish organic impairment such as dementia from functional, e.g. depression, because although slow at first depressives tend to improve their performance with the repetition of information as the test continues, whereas the demented do not.

The Inglis Paired Associates Learning Test measures the number of times it takes subjects to learn the unlikely association between three pairs of words, e.g. Cabbage—Pen, Knife—Chimney, Sponge—Trumpet. This is a sensitive test of memory disorder in the elderly, and a useful discriminator between depressive and organic impairment.

The Bender Gestalt Test measures another important function than intelligence and memory—the ability to make sense of what is seen. Two designs are to be copied, and scores are based on the accuracy of the reproduction.

The Digit Copying Test measures speed of response—the number of digits copied in two minutes.

Psychological testing is complementary to clinical appraisal. The psychologist can map out the patient's disabilities more precisely than can the psychiatrist at an ordinary clinical interview and may discern more subtle disabilities than those simply affecting memory. Sometimes he can help to localise an area of abnormality; for example, a marked disparity between the ability to learn visually rather than by ear suggests a lesion of the temporal lobe.

The psychologist also quantifies his findings and by successive testing can show in what ways there is any improvement or deterioration. Dementia scales which are simple instruments for more general use, have a similar purpose. The Gresham is in four sections concerning orientation in time and space, memory for personal events, past and recent, general knowledge and the lay-out of the ward. A total score of less than 35 is likely to be morbid. The scale described by Blessed (1968) asks questions of a close informant about changes in the past six months, competence in personal, domestic and social activities and changes in habits, personality, interest and drive. Silver's test (1972) contains a simple questionnaire testing memory, vocabulary, calculation, orientation and speech and practical tests with matchsticks and toys. Scores of less than 30 (out of 45) are usually inconsistent with independence at home.

If there is ever to be a remedy for dementia it is likely only to be effective in the early stages, while it is possible that family support in the community may be continued longer or more often for good if counselling and practical help are given sooner rather than later. But *early dementia*, which rarely comes the way of the psychiatrist is difficult to diagnose with any certainty. In 1979 Sir Martin Roth wrote: 'we are very poor at recognising dementia in its early stages. In our own community studies we failed to recognise four fifths of those who were to present with unequivocal dementia four to five years later, but in other cases in which a positive diagnosis was made it was proved erroneous'.

The Duke University studies (Gianturco & Busse, 1978) of elderly volunteers, year by year, have shown that the course of what appears to be mild dementia is highly variable, with remissions and exacerbations. Even more severe cases of supposed dementia are not infrequently misdiagnosed. Thus in follow-up studies of patients with (mainly) pre-senile (i.e. before the age of 65) dementia referred to a neurological department, Marsden & Harrison (1972) found 22 (21 per cent) of 106 patients not to be demented but suffering other psychiatric illness, chiefly depression, and of those at first diagnosed as demented in psychiatric departments. Nott &

Fleminger (1975) traced 35 (of 50) patients later and found less than half to be demented, while Ron et al (1979) followed up 51 of 52 patients admitted to the Bethlem Royal and Maudsley Hospitals five to 15 years later and rejected the original diagnosis in 16 (31 per cent).

There is, then, no room for complacency about diagnosing dementia. The experts are those who know how fallible they can be. There is a great need to sharpen clinical acumen by careful observation and follow up studies. The possibility should be carefully considered whenever an older person is having problems, e.g. attending the surgery or out patients, in hospital, seeking extra services at home, a move to sheltered housing or a place in a Home. All the evidence should be weighed, and if doubt remains there should be a review in six months time. It is to be hoped that one day there will be a practical reliable biochemical test to indicate the onset of, say, Alzheimer's disease, but as yet no tests, be they biochemical, psychological, physiological or radiological can be regarded as adequate substitutes for the painstaking history and mental state examination, especially where the latter is extended to include the dwelling as well as the person who lives in it.

There is as yet little evidence that any *treatment* arrests the progress of Alzheimer's disease or multi-infarct dementia. Vitamins will not help unless there is malnutrition aggravating the effects of the dementia and even then will not check the basic disorder. Their value is largely that of giving the patient's family (and perhaps the doctor too) the comfort that something is being done. However, increasing the output of a failing heart by giving digoxin and diuretics, correcting any anaemia and controlling infection will help the dementing brain to use its residual capacity to the full. In hypertensive sufferers from multi-infarct dementia lowering the blood pressure is too late; while it might reduce the wear and tear on the arteries, it is more likely to reduce the blood supply to the brain through vessels narrowed by atheroma. While vascular surgery to the internal carotid artery (which runs up through the neck to supply the brain) has relieved some important neurological consequences of narrowing or obliteration of that vessel, it is rarely successful where there is dementia because this nearly always means widespread damage to the smaller cerebral vessels too. Anticoagulants are very occasionally indicated, where dementia (or more often a sub-acute delirium) is due to emboli from a clot in a fibrillating left auricle, but not where there is extensive arterial disease.

It must in all honesty be recognised that the vast majority of those who appear to be demented at the initial assessment will prove to be so subsequently. Any hypothyroidism, B12 or folate deficiency, or positive seriology indicating neurosyphilis will probably be coincidental, or at least their treatment will have little effect on the severity or the course of the dementia.

A useful review of *drugs for dementia*, variously claimed to be cerebral vasodilators or cerebral activators, appeared in the *Drugs and Therapeutics Bulletin* in 1975, and concluded that while some seemed in the laboratory to have some action on the brain or its blood supply, none could be recommeded for routine use. None have been shown significantly to improve the daily living activities, which matter most. Yesavage (1979) noted that significantly more controlled studies showed benefit from drugs supposed to improve the metabolism of neurones (dihydroergotamine mesylate, naftidrofuryl) than from those supposed to have a vasodilator action only (cyclandelate, isoxsuprine). But the possible benefits of such drugs are small, they are costly and not without side effects and problems of compliance are so great that their main value may again be a placebo effect on the supporters and attendants. As yet no remedies based on the acetyl choline deficiency theory of Alzheimer's disease (see above) such as choline chloride, choline bitartrate and lecithin (phosphatidyl choline) have proved effective, or, in the case of physostigmine, which has some intriguing short term effects but has to be given intravenously, practical. There are reasonable hopes that further research along these lines may prove rewarding (Kendall, 1979) but an imminent breakthrough seems unlikely.

A *psychological*, educational approach, however, seems to have something to offer now. Folsom (1967) in the United States advocated *reality orientation therapy*, a technique for teaching demented subjects some simple, basic facts about time, place and persons around them and the names and uses of commonly encountered objects. Subjects learn, relearn and are stimulated into repeatedly using this information. Formal daily classes are complemented by staff who reiterate such information if the patient is in institutional care. 'Good morning, Mrs Green. I'm Nurse Jones. Here we are in Wellington Ward in St Ann's Hospital in Bridport. Its a cloudy day, it looks like rain. Would you like some breakfast? Let's find the dining room'. Needless to say, this is not a monologue by the nurse: the patient is encouraged to repeat what has just been said and to respond.

The techniques of reality orientation therapy are well described by Holden & Woods (1982), while the studies by Brooke et al (1975) and Woods (1979) have demonstrated that for teaching forgetful old people a few useful facts ROT is not rot! The best subjects are those with features of early multi-infarct or 'benign' dementia with well preserved personalities and intact language.

More speculative is the use of reminiscence aids and nostalgia techniques which exploit Ribot's law (the tendency of the demented to recall the past more clearly than the present) to evoke that past and by reminding them who they were to help them regain awareness of who they are. Old songs, sounds, photos and materials, even smells are used, usually in a group setting.

In general *management* rather than treatment is the approach appropriate to dementia, and the main objective is to keep the patient in his or her own home for as long as possible, provided that neither she nor those caring for her suffer unduly. Quite apart from the fact that there is only a limited amount of institutional care available, it is obvious that a confused old person will be less at a loss in familiar surroundings. To achieve this objective, the *social* aspects of dementia must be recognised.

The 20 per cent of demented patients who are in institutions are not simply the most confused. Admission is rarely sought simply because of the severity of the disorder, but usually when there is a social crisis involving the key supporter. A devoted husband may himself have been admitted to hospital with an acute illness, a helpful neighbour rehoused, or an attentive daughter, confronted by her husband's resentment, an ailing child or her own depression, be no longer able to cope.

It has already been remarked above that the poor and the isolated are most likely to be admitted to mental hospital with dementia. The stigma will drive most middle-class families to make other arrangements, such as nursing home or private nurse, for their demented elderly. Devoted couples are unlikely to be separated by dementia; indeed as had been previously stated, some husbands find a raison d'etre after retirement in caring for an ailing wife. Close-knit families, especially in areas (like the East End of London) where they continue to live near to each other, will go to great lengths to keep their confused parents at home. On the other hand old people isolated by bereavement, distance from friends and family or alienating personality traits are more likely to be referred for institutional care. Often it seems that very large familes cope less readily with their aged parents tham smaller, probably because the children had a less close individual relationship with their parents in childhood. On the whole it appears that parents who gave their children a lot of love get it back from them in later life: 'Cast they bread upon the waters; for thou shalt find it after many days.'

To keep the patients at home, *support* for those relatives, friends or neighbours chiefly concerned should be organised as soon as the diagnosis of dementia is made. This support, for which the general practitioner and the Social Services Department are especially responsible, though voluntary workers and other relatives (see p. 186) may be involved, should be moral and material.

Moral support includes explanation of the nature of dementia, its probable course and the eventual outcome, which should be discussed as honestly as it has been set out in this chapter; enlightenment about the sometimes painfully bewildering change in personality, and irrational outbursts; encouragement; and a deal of sympathetic listening. It is necessary to recognise how excessive anxiety, guilt, overprotectiveness and anger may be aroused in families and friends, in order to aid the expression of these feelings and give proper counsel. Otherwise eventually the depression and sense of futility, when prolonged, painstaking care is repaid only with the inevitable worsening of the patient's condition, will lead to rejection. Support needs to take account of the realities of the situation, not only when the burden has clearly become too great and a respite is needed, but also when the old person is unwittingly being made a scapegoat for other problems in the family which need to be dealt with in their own right, e.g. inadequate housing, or a disturbed child. Support is not a matter of a single visit for exhortation, or sporadic looking in, but of regular, reliable contact.

Practical support includes the provision, where appropriate, of a home help, Meals on Wheels and day care (at a day hospital or local authority day centre), all of which maintain the isolated patient or enable the key supporter to have time off for work or recreation. Bergmann et al (1978) concluded that such help, if not freely available to all should be given first to those with supportive but potentially strained families, to enable them to carry on. Demented old people living alone, unless they have unusual insight, are decidedly more likely to require institutional care in the end anyway. Baker & Byrne (1977) made extensive use of day hospitals and centres for the demented and claimed that the need for continuing hospital care was thus much reduced but many, e.g. Jolley (1977), would contest this. Many day hospitals in Britain are simply containing demented old people who certainly need continuing institutional care until a place becomes available (Greene & Timbury, 1979). The Department of Health & Social Security in Britain (which leads most other countries in its development of day care) has recommended that there should be two or three places for demented patients in day hospitals for every thousand people over

65. The help of a district or community psychiatrc nurse, health visitor, bathing attendant, warden (either for an estate or a special sheltered housing development), 'sitter in' (if these are to be found anywhere) an incontinent laundry service, and (holiday) admission to hospital or an old people's home all ease the burden. An attendance allowance occasionally strengthens the supporter's resolve to keep the old person at home—not for mercenary reasons, but because it may be hard to make ends meet when one has a relative so dependent that one cannot go out to work. The use of a 'good neighbours' scheme, where suitable, interested neighbours are paid to give their care regularly, may ensure aid for the isolated. The provision of a commode, and advice about taking the patients to the lavatory regularly, especially after meals, reduce incontinence. An outside bolt on doors to the outside reduces wandering. And complaints that the gas is left on unlit may be dealt with by seeing that it is turned off at the main when the patient is unattended or even the provision of an electric cooker (which costs the country a lot less than taking the patient into care).

Inevitably in the course of dementia the patient becomes *unfit to handle her affairs*. Sometimes this disability is of major importance, as when the pension is not collected, rent and accounts are unpaid and threats of eviction and other legal action follows. The more affluent the patient, the greater the anxiety. A power of attorney is rarely appropriate as dementia prevents the patient from knowing what she is doing when she gives this power to another. Instead the proper agency to approach in England is the Official Solicitor at the Court of Protection (through a solicitor or the Personal Applications Branch, Straffordshire House, Store Street, London WC1), who, on receiving medical confirmation of the patient's incompetence will either administer her affairs or appoint a trustworthy relative or occasionally a social worker to do so. If supplementary benefit is being paid arrangements may be made to deduct, e.g. rent money at source.

Sedation should be used very sparingly. It is too easy to turn a fit, if confused, old person into a dry and drowsy one. However, the judicious use of the phenothiazine tranquillisers in low dosage may lessen agitation, wandering and hostility. Promazine (Sparine) has a very mild action; its popularity is attributable to the rarity of side effects and, perhaps, a placebo effect on those who give it. The feeling that something is being done may be of comfort, and alter attitudes, even though that something is very little indeed. Chlorpromazine (Largactil) is more useful, but may lower the blood pressure and cause faintness. Thioridazine (Melleril) has an activity intermediate between that of Sparine and Largactil, and is relatively free from side effects. This and haloperidol (Serenace) are the most generally useful tranquillisers for the restless demented patient. Haloperidol calms without unduly sedating, but may cause Parkinsonism and muscle spasms, which may then have to be treated with an anti-Parkinsonian drug like orphenadrine (Disipal). Benzodiazepines such as diazepam (Valium), are of little value, but chlormethiazole (Heminevrin) which has a relatively short action is a useful alternative. In many patients unfortunately tranquillisers and sedatives tend to have an all or nothing effect, the patient being either untouched or knocked out: it is all too easy thus to turn a psychogeriatric into a geriatric problem.

Sustained distress and depression in the setting of dementia requires relief (if possible) as much as does physical pain. Mostly tricyclic antidepressants (e.g. amitryptyline, dothiepin) are prescribed, but I must confess that I freqnently find amphetamine (in the form of Dexedrine) more useful, and the risk of habituation in a demented old person is unimportant.

Hypnotics are sometimes necessary, but care must be taken not to sedate the patient to such an extent that she is drowsy and 'hung over' next day to wake fighting fit for bedtime. Chloral is tried and true—as the hydrate, in a draught, or as dichloralphenazone (Welldorm) tablets. Nitrazepam (Mogadon) is the sleeping tablet most widely used by the elderly, but has a rather long action, for which reason shorter acting benzodiazepimes like triazolam (Halcion) and temazepam (Euhypnos, Normison) or the chemically quite different chlormethiazole (Heminevrin) are often to be preferred (for doses of these drugs see Ch. 14).

If, despite all these measures, though, the point is reached where the patient has become a danger to herself, or the family are sorely stressed, *institutional care* should be provided as speedily as possible. This is more likely to be achieved if the psychiatist, geriatrician or welfare officer has been previously made aware of the patient, preferably by a domiciliary assessment. Even at this stage, care may not be long-term. There may be an improvement in the patient's condition (especially where the dementia is vascular), the relatives may feel like taking up the load again after having a break or the hospital or old people's home may be able to deploy a wider range of community resources than had been used previously. Where there is a psychogeriatric assessment unit (Ch. 12) the first admission is likely to be there. Only very restless, destructive, aggressive and (possibly) doubly incontinent patients require long-term care in a psychiatric ward; the Department of Health estimates that 2·5 to 3 hospital beds should be made available for this purpose for every thousand people over 65. Demented patients who are also ill and/or unable to walk should go to a geriatric ward. Otherwise fit demented patients who can no longer live at home belong in old people's homes—the part three accommodation provided by the local authorities, or voluntary. Some areas have special homes for the elderly mentally infirm (EMI) which are needed most for the demented.

Where institutional care is needed the inability to meet that need because the accommodation is not at present available creates a serious problem for giving proper care and maintaining morale. The social services or the psychogeriatric team may be embarrassed to appear to condone a delay which they deplore. Such delays are probably unfortunately commoner in ageing, indigent Britain than in some other countries like Scandinavia and North America which have put more of their resources into institutions (admittedly, often at some cost to community care).

Especially in institutions, sedation should not be used too freely. Drugs are a poor substitute for exercise and occupation. It should be recognised that old people do not require much more than 5 or 6 hours' sleep at night (though they may like to cat-nap by day), and that the 14 hours they spend in bed at a stretch in many establishments are for the staff's convenience, not the patients'. Oversedation is one cause of excessive incontinence in an old people's home or ward, and also contributes to falls. I have often heard it argued that patients must be put to bed before the night staff come on duty, because there are more day than night staff, but it cannot be regarded as good practice to start tucking everyone in straight after a 4 o'clock tea. I have even heard it owned (doubtless with tongue in cheek) that the patients must be made to have their sleep so that the night nurse can get hers—the poor girl has been working all day in her other job. I am afraid that where there are staff shortages this situation is not altogether unknown, but it can hardly be condoned.

Once institutional care is established, *respect* for the resident or patient as a person, allowing her to have some personal possessions and as far as possible to wear her own clothes, to have plenty of space, exercise, a regular regime with some form of simple occupation, unrestricted visiting, and a tolerant, understanding sufficient staff with a good sense of humour help to make the final months or years as pleasant as possible Occupational therapy and sometimes speech therapy may lessen dependency and mitigate the manifestations of dementia and can do a great deal for morale of staff as well as patients. The physiotherapist helps the staff to keep their charges fit and active. Open visiting enables families to continue to share the care of the old member, easing the pain and guilt that are often experienced after handing the task over to others, and helping the staff out too.

As yet conditions in many institutions are far from ideal (though rarely as bad as depicted in sensational publications such as *Sans Everything*) and shortages of staff and amenities mean that too often little more is given than basic care. However it is to be hoped that the greater awareness of needs reflected in the Department of Health's current concern for the elderly and the mentally ill will be reflected in better education, improved attitudes, greater expenditure and much wider provision of the best kind of care.

It is important that staff see their role in the context of the whole range of services available to the elderly. Dementia is not always a living death, and many patients are capable of leading contented lives if given the opportunity and proper care. Euthanasia would be quite inappropriate for such old people who need not be seen as miserable and expendable just because their memories fail them. On the other hand there are those whose vacant wretchedness is not worth prolonging, who should usually be allowed to die of whatever potentially fatal illesss (usually pneumonia) may develop, with no more treatment than is needed to keep them comfortable. The decision to withhold more active treatment (such as an antibiotic) is ultimately the doctor's, but should be taken after consultation with any relatives and the ward staff.

Incidently, whereas Roth noted in 1955 that 60 per cent of those with the diagnosis of senile psychosis died within six months of admission to hospital, and 80 per cent within two years, my findings in my own hospital 24 years later are very different (Table 2).

This shows a mean survival time of 23 months (17 for men 27 for women) while 32 per cent of men and no less than 50 per cent of women survived over 2 years. My figures exclude assessment and holiday admissions and refer only to old people admitted after some

Table 2 Survival of elderly dements admitted to the London Hospital (St Clement's) for continuing care from January 1974 – October 1977

Survival	3 months	3–6 months	6 months – 1 year	1–2 years	2–3 years	3–4 years	4–5 years	5 years	Totals
Maie	6(27%)	—	5(23%)	4(18%)	3(14%)	3(14%)	—	1(5%)	22(100%)
Female	3(10%)	1(3%)	6(20%)	5(17%)	4(13%)	4(13%)	4(13%)	3(10%)	30(100%)
All	9(17%)	1(2%)	11(21%)	9(17%)	7(14%)	7(14%)	4(8%)	4(8%)	52(100%)

delay, for continuing care, so they may not be strictly comparable with Roth's. Most had definitely been demented for several years before admission and may have indicated their hardiness by surviving to be admitted. However, the indication is that with a reasonable proportion to staff to patients or residents, good care and a life of some quality the demented may survive in institutions far longer than planners have realised. The dilemma is obvious: while they remain their places cannot be taken, and better care may well mean more problems for the demented patient in the community. Nevertheless, in far too many institutions care is very basic, staff have small vocation for their arduous work, and life for the residents is a drab demeaning routine. There is still enormous scope for improvement and with the concern of governments, the development of such professional bodies (in Britain) as the Section for the Psychiatry of Old Age, the British Geriatric Society, the Health Advisory Service, the Royal College of Nursing and special interest groups among social workers, and the energy and outspokenness of such voluntary organisations as Age Concern, Mind and the National Corporation for the Care of Old People, it is likely that progress will continue.

REFERENCES

Albert M 1979 Subcortical dementia. In: Katzman R, Terry R (eds) Alzheimer's disease, senile dementia and related disorders. Raven Press, New York

Alzheimer A 1907 Über eine eigenartige Erkrankung der Hirnrinde. Allg Z Psychiat 64: 146

Baker A A, Byrne R J F 1977 Another syle of psychogeriatric service. Brit J Psychiat 130: 123

Bergmann K, Foster E M, Justice A W, Matthews V 1978 Management of the demented patient in the community. Brit J Psychiat 132: 441

Blessed G, Tomlinson B E, Roth M 1968 The association between quantitative measures of dementia and of degenerative changes in the cerebral grey matter of elderly subjects. Brit J Psychiat 114: 797

Brooke P, Degun G, Mather M 1975 Reality orientation, a treatment for psychogeriatric patients: a controlled study. Brit J Psychiat 127: 42

Corsellis, J A N 1962 Mental Illness and the Ageing Brain. Maudsley Monograph No 9 London: Oxford University Press.

Davies P, Maloney A J F 1976 Selective loss of central cholinergic neurones in Alzheimer's disease. Lancet 2: 1403

Department of Health and Social Security 1972 Services for Mental Illness Related to Old Age HM(72)71

Drugs and Therapeutics Bulletin 1975 Drugs for dementia 13: 85

Folsom J C 1976 Intensive hospital therapy for psychogeriatric patients. Curr Psychiat Ther 7: 209

Gianturco D T, Busse E W 1978 Psychiatric problems encountered during a long term study of normal ageing volunteers. In Isaacs A D, Post F (eds) Studies in Geriatric Psychiatry. Wiley, Chichester

Greene J G, Timbury G C 1979 A Geriatric Psychiatry Day Hospital Service: a 5 year review. Age and Ageing 8: 49

Hare, M 1978 Clinical check list for diagnosis of dementia. Brit Med J 2: 226
Holden U, Woods R 1982 Reality orientation therapy. Churchill Livingstone, Edinburgh
Jacoby A, Levy R, Dawson J M 1980 Computerised Tomography in the Elderly.
  1. The Normal Population. Brit J Psychiat 136: 249
  2. Senile Dementia: Diagnosis and functional impairment. Brit J Psychiat 136: 256
Jolley D 1977 Hospital in patient provision for patients with dementia. Brit Med J 1: 1335
Kallman F J 1951 Comparative adaptational social and psychometric date on life histories of senescent twin pairs. Amer J Hum Gener 3: 65
Kay D W K, Bergmann K Foster E M, McKechnie A A, Roth M 1970 Mental illness and hospital usage in the elderly: a random sample followed up. Compr Psychiat 2: 1
Kendall M J 1979 Will drugs help patients with Alzheimer's disease? Age and Ageing 8: 86
Kral V A 1965 The senile amnestic syndrome. In Psychiatric disorders in the aged. W P Symposium, Geigy, Manchester
Larsson T, Sjogren T, Jacobsen G 1963 Senile dementia. Acta psychiat Scand, 39 suppl 167
Lipanski Z 1980 A new look at organic brain syndromes. Am J Psychiat 137: 674
Lishman W A (ed) 1977 Senile and presenile dementias. Medical Research Council, London
Marsden C D 1978 The diagnosis of dementia. In Isaacs A D, Post F (eds) Studies in geriatric psychiatry, Wiley, Chichester
Marsden C D, Harrison M J D 1972 Outcome of investigations of patients with presenile dementia. Brit Med J 1: 249
McDonald C 1968 Clinical heterogeneity in senile dementia. Brit J Psychiat 115: 267
Nott P N, Fleminger J J 1975 Presenile dementia: the difficulties of early diagnosis. Acta psychiat Scand 51: 210
Olsen M I, Shaw M 1969 Presenile dementia and Alzheimer's disease in Mongolism. Brain 92: 147
Perry E K, Perry R H, Blessed G, Tomlinson B E 1977 Necropsy evidence of central cholinergic deficits in senile dementia. Lancet 1: 189
Post F 1962 The Significance of Affective Symptoms in Old Age. Maudsley Monograph No. 10 Oxford University Press, London
Ron M A, Toone B K, Garralda M A, Lishman W A 1979 Diagnostic accuracy in presenile dementia. Brit J Psychiat 134: 161
Roth M 1955 The natural history of mental disorder in old age. J Ment Sci 101: 281
Roth M 1979 Introduction to Positive approaches to mental infirmity in elderly people. 1978 Annual Conference Report, Mind, London.
Roth M, Myers D H 1969 The diagnosis of dementia. Brit J Hosp Med 2: 705
Silver C P 1972 Simple methods of testing ability in geriatric patients. Geront clin 14: 110
Woods R T 1979 Reality orientation and staff attention in a controlled study. Brit J Psychiat 134: 502
Yesavage J A 1979 Vasodilators in senile dementia. Arch Gen Psychiat 36: 220

FURTHER READING

Alzheimer's Disease. Glen A I M, Whalley L J 1980 Churchill Livingstone, Edinburgh
Cowan, Daphne, Wright, Patricia. Gourlay, A J, Smith A, Barron G, De Gruchy J,
Copeland J R M, Kelleher M J, Kellett J M 1975 A comparative psychometric assessment of psychogeriatric and geriatric patients. Brit J Psychiat 127: 33
Dementia in old age 1979 Office of Health Economics. White Crescent, Luton
Lishman W A 1978 Organic Psychiatry. Blackwell, London

7

Depression

'Know syphilis, and you know medicine; know depression', it has been said, 'and you know psychiatry'. This is especially true of depressive illness arising in old age.

Depression is of course a normal emotion, the natural response to loss and disappointment, just as anxiety is to insecurity and the threat of danger. Like the inflammation which accompanies healing and the fever which is part of the body's defence against infection, depression is an essential feature of *mourning*, the mental work we must do to divest ourselves of something we have valued, and carry on living without it. Depression is only abnormal (or *pathological*) when out of proportion, in intensity or duration, or both, to any stress which might have given rise to it; indeed, the so-called *endogenous* depression is a state of deep melancholy unrelated to any obvious loss at all.

At all ages, from adolescence onwards, depression is the commonest psychiatric illness. And despite the importance of organic disorders in old age, depression is almost twice as common as dementia. Various *factors predispose* to depression. *Heredity* is important, especially in younger patients; there is a family history of depressive illness (or mania) in 80 per cent of those becoming severely depressed before the age of 50, and in 44 per cent of those developing the disorder after 65. A significant proportion of depressives are *children of broken homes*, or were *bereaved* of a parent in early life. The typical *personality* liable to depression in old age is *obsessional*, serious, conscientious, thorough, rigid, introverted and unable to display aggression.

Purely *physical* stresses can *precipitate* depression—infections, especially virus, e.g. influenza, and certain drugs, such as steroids and rauwolfia, which was useful for dropping the blood pressure in hypertensives but was abandoned because of the danger of inducing deep, even suicidal depression.

By far the most important cause of depression in the elderly, though, is *psychological stress*. The various *losses* discussed in

Chapter 2 all dispose to depression, and account for its increased frequency in old age. The greatest stress of all is the loss of a spouse. An accumulation of life events, most of them lesser, has been found significantly often to precede the onset of depressive illness (Brown & Harris, 1978). However, *frustrated aggression* can also cause depression, and in late life this occurs most often between couples stuck with each other and angry or resentful but unable to quarrel; then, it seems, the aggression which cannot be expressed outwardly is turned inwards, so that the depression is partly to be explained as hostility against the self.

The most extreme form of such hostility is, of course, *suicide*. The highest suicide rate is in the elderly, especially in men. In comparison with younger suicides, fewer of the older are of unstable personality, and more, indeed the majority, are suffering from depressive illness. Sadly, a study by Barraclough (1971) showed that most of a group of elderly depressives who killed themselves had suffered from their depression for only about 6 months (and were therefore potentially more recoverable than those referred to psychiatrists, who have on average been ill for over a year) and most had seen their doctor a week before their death, but few were receiving treatment for their depression.

The experiments of Seligman (1975) suggest that depression sometimes represents a *learned state of helplessness*, in which the subject has reached the dismal conclusion that whatever he does he cannot influence the unpleasant situation in which he finds himself. This is, of course, far too often the lot of the elderly, especially when in institutions.

Despite the patient's frequently adverse circumstances, depression is the most treatable of all psychogeriatric illnesses. Yet far too often it goes unrecognised, and if the consequence is not aften as serious as suicide, many lives are needlessly blighted by prolonged misery. The detection and successful treatment of depressive illness are among the particular rewards of geriatric psychiatry.

There is a long-standing controversy in psychiatry over whether there are, essentially, *one* or *two* forms of depression. One school (Lewis, 1971) holds that depression is a single illness with two extremes: at one end the patient whose condition is almost entirely due to circumstances, at the other one whose depressive constitution is almost wholly responsible, and most patients lie somewhere between the two. The other school (Carney, Roth & Garside, 1965) claims that there are two kinds of depressive illness (labelled respectively endogenous and reactive) roughly corresponding to the two extremes postulated by the first school, but fundamentally different in nature—affecting different personalities, running a different course, and responding differently to treatment. While statistical evidence favours the views of the second school, I shall attempt in this chapter to avoid commitment to either side by describing depression under the simple headings of severe and milder.

SEVERE DEPRESSION

While severe depression is frequently (though not invariably) precipitated by stress, for example, bereavement, the mood change goes far beyond what can be considered as normal. The misery is intense, sustained and related to all aspects of life, not only to what has been lost. There is a sense of deep *despair*. At the least, life will be seen as not worth living, and the patient may admit that he would be glad to go to sleep and never wake. And at a stage beyond this, he is actively suicidal, feeling that there is nothing to hold him to life and, indeed, that he is unfit to live. Characteristically, though, the depression is at its worst in the morning (when many of us, even if free from depression, are not at our best) and lightens towards evening. So marked may this *diurnal variation* of mood be that it can be misleading in assessing the patient's mood to see him at different times of different days.

The depression is usually accompanied by enormous *guilt*, which is never justified by past or present behaviour and may be frankly delusional. In its mildest form this is manifest in a feeling of 'not belonging' and of being unfit for company. A common notion in depressed elderly women is that they have not the right clothing for any occasion, and I have heard this argued vehemently as the reason for not coming into hospital or having ECT. Ideas of *unworthiness* may be vigorously expressed: 'I'm not fit to be in hospital. You ought to put me up against a wall and shoot me.' 'I'm in Hell—and that's where I belong'. *Delusions* along these lines may be quite bizarre, such as a conviction of personal responsibility for whatever disaster —floods, earthquakes, war—is currently in the news. One old lady, who regarded herself as a sort of Jonah, was certain that she was responsible for the presence of the other one and a half thousand patients in the psychiatric hospital where she was being treated, and that it was because of her that I had more grey hairs every time she saw me! Such delusions are often accompanied by *auditory hallucinations*—voices which disparage and abuse the patient: 'She's dirty. She smells. She's a whore!'—and with whose judgements the patient is inclined to agree. There may be *paranoid* beliefs that most people know, disapprove of and comment critically on the patient's disgrace. However, in contrast to paraphrenia, the patient, though distressed by these imagined criticisms, is usually not aggrieved, feeling that they are justified.

Elderly men, in particular, may have ideas of *poverty*. These sometimes have their origins in anxieties about how to manage on a retirement pension, and especially in fears of not being able to meet demands for income tax. Ruin, even imprisonment, seem virtual certainties, and no amount of explanation about the adequacy of financial resources gives reassurance. A few such patients doubt their entitlement to a pension at all, and in fact lead a life so frugal that they starve.

Starvation is also a serious consequence of the extreme and extraordinary *hypochondriasis* which characterises severe depressive states. Constipation is a common accompaniment of depression and may give rise to the belief that the bowels have seized up altogether. Food is supposed to be rotting inside the body, or to form a solid mass from the throat to the rectum, spilling over into the body's cavities. The *loss of appetite* and *weight* usual in depression are then intensified until there is complete refusal of food and fluids, with danger to life from dehydration and emaciation. This situation is a psychiatric emergency requiring urgent treatment (i.e. today, not after the weekend). A similar delusion is that no urine is being passed, and consequently the intake of water is restricted. Demonstration to the patient that he is passing water is dismissed. It seems that the 'image' of grossly disturbed bodily function is more real to him than what his body is actually doing. Various other hypochondriacal fears include those of losing hair, and of being lousy.

The *behaviour* accompanying the deep depression and these dire thoughts is of two contrasting kinds. A few show *retardation*, a striking slowing-up of thought and action. There is no spontaneous speech, answers are monosyllabic and long-delayed, or the patient may be completely mute. Similarly there is little or no physical activity, the patient being sunk in the deepest gloom, his face registering only blank misery; in depressive stupor there is complete immobility, and the patient wets and soils where he sits, and easily develops bedsores.

The contrasted form of behaviour, more typical of the elderly depressive, *is agitation*. Even more marked than the depression is extreme restless anxiety, the patient endlessly pacing up and down, grabbing the skirts or lapels of passers-by and begging for reassurance which cannot, however, be accepted. Sensing, perhaps the irritation which such behaviour eventually arouses (and even while they understand, staff, let alone relatives, can find such importunate distress very trying) the patient may resort to histrionics, or grossly *hysterical* activity, in order more vividly to communicate his depression. Unfortunately the effect may be quite the opposite: the 'hysteria' is dismissed as attention-seeking, and the patient as a phoney. It needs to be said that 'hysteria' in the elderly always has a serious basis, and that those patients who clamour for attention so urgently usually need it. Agitated depressives are the most suicidal.

Disturbances of appetite and bowel function have already been mentioned. *Sleep* is also impaired. Characteristically there is less difficulty in falling than in remaining asleep. *Early morning waking* is absolutely typical, at 3 or 4 a.m., at which hour the patient feels at his very lowest.

(It is not unlikely that severe depressives were prominent among those hapless old people, who, two or three hundred years ago, were accused of witchcraft. The marked change from the usual personality could well suggest demoniacal possession to a superstitious populace, and none would be likely to have made more vigorous accusation than the patient herself. Very probably her wish to be punished, rather than treated, and to be removed painfully from the face of the earth was all too readily granted.)

Milder Depression
This is a far less dramatic disorder, with less distinctive features, and hence easily overlooked or attributed to normal ageing. Nevertheless, it matters because life is rendered dreary, or fraught with anxiety, and treatment can be effective.

The contrast between whatever stresses there may be (such as the disability of arthritis or bronchitis) and the degree of depression is less apparent, but the depression is still disproportionate if one considers how much better many old people react to very similar problems.

There are *two* main forms of milder depression in the elderly, roughly corresponding to the retarded and the agitated varieties of severe depression.

The first form might conveniently be described as *apathetic* depression. Loss of former interests, particularly social, is noteworthy. It is too much of an effort to go out and about and meet people. There is a tendency to sit indoors, moping. The papers are not read, the television loses its attractions, the wireless is ignored. Friends are shunned not because they are no longer liked (though they may get that impression), but because conversation has become an ordeal. There is increasing withdrawal, even to bed, and a measure of self-neglect, though this is rarely serious.

Anxiety is the main feature of the other kind of milder depression, and this is mainly manifest as *hypochondriasis*. This, lacking the bizarre quality of the delusions about the body's functioning in severe depression, is likely to be taken more literally by the doctor. The patient worries about his head, his heart and his bowels. He fears cancer, or simply that he is going to collapse, or pass out. Complaints of dizziness, ringing in the ears, burning in the throat and the abdomen, difficulty in swallowing, fullness, wind, diarrhoea or constipation, pains in the chest, side or down the legs, backache, 'funny feelings down below', itching, numbness or tingling are commonplace. Thorough investigations fail to detect an adequate physical cause. Inevitably, abnormalities are occasionally turned up, but their treatment gives no relief to the symptoms. These are demanding patients, who call out the doctor unnecessarily, in his opinion, and haunt casualty departments. They are referred from one specialist to another, neither giving the satisfaction of response to treatment, nor gaining that of being cured. They turn to other agents than doctors—friends, family and neighbours, social workers and priests—to be met at first with consideration, but later, as they appear unhelped by energetic ministrations and their demands continue, with annoyance. They feel, and are felt to be, a nuisance; but they were not always so.

The mood of the milder depressive is not always one of actual misery, but may simply consist of an incapacity for enjoyment. Many, however, are actively unhappy, and are easily upset and made to weep. Any *variation* of mood through the day takes the form of feeling more weary and wretched in the evening rather than on waking. There is also variation from day to day, with brief spells, sometimes, of complete respite, but the depression is never absent for longer than a week. Guilt is rarely a feature of milder depression. Instead *irritability* and peevishness are common, mainly towards a long-suffering daughter or spouse. Though the intense *phobias* so frequent in younger patients are inconspicuous, *anxiety* may be expressed as an actual fear of going out of doors (not merely a reluctance), as well as in hypochondriasis. The patient is more susceptible to 'cheering up' than the severe depressive, and may rise briefly to a social occasion if coaxed or gently bullied to participate, but without such stimulation rapidly subsides into her dejection.

A loss of *energy* accompanies the lack of interest, and may be pronounced enough to suggest a physical cause for debility, such as anaemia. *Appetite* may be impaired, with weight loss of usually no more than a stone (9–10 kg) in the course of several months, or increased: over-eating is at all ages a common compensation for unhappiness, and far more people 'cry' than 'laugh—and grow fat'. Difficulty with *sleep* is in falling asleep; the patient lies awake worrying—as often as not, about not sleeping!

The milder states of depression are very uncommon in the psychiatric ward, but occur frequently elsewhere—in general and geriatric wards, old people's homes, day centres and hospitals, outpatient clinics and the community at large. They are far commoner, indeed, than severe depression, though the exact incidence is hard to determine as they are less well defined. However, a survey in Newcastle showed the total *prevalence* of affective (emotional) illness and neurosis in those over 65 to be 26 per cent, and the great majority were in the milder category.

The following fairly typical *case history* illustrates the main features of milder depression:

Mrs Brown, aged 73, lived with her second husband in a comfortable old terraced house in a surprisingly quiet cul-de-sac in the East End. She had been unwell 'this time' for about a month: 'As soon as I drink anything I come over all burning, all round me stomach and up me side and back. I sweat terrible. I ain't got a bit of energy. If anyone comes to see me I lose me voice'. She could not get to sleep without sleeping tablets. Over the last year her weight had dropped by a stone. She had no interest in food or anything else, and could not enjoy life. She had not left the house for the past month. She felt at her lowest, her husband said, at the end of the day. There were days of relative well being.

It turned out that this was merely the latest bout of a disorder which had troubled her for at least six years, if not ten, and was increasingly disabling. Ten years ago she had had her gallbladder removed, and she felt that she had not been quite right since then, being subject to bouts of weakness. She had been worse for the past six years. Her husband had retired three years ago, and for the past year had done all the housework, cooking and shopping; neither seemed to mind.

She was a twin, one of nine children. An elder sister had died recently, and it seemed likely that this had precipitated the present bout. The patient's identical twin sister lived in a new town, and also had 'nerve trouble'. Her childhood was happy. Her father died when she was 15, her mother at 72. After working in tailoring she first married at 20. Her husband, who went out and drunk a lot, died of 'heart trouble' in 1937. They got on, because she was too busy with their three children to quarrel. These children were now all married, none lived far away, and she saw them all once a fortnight. One was in the East End, where she herself had always lived.

There were no children by the second husband, who had not been previously married. Before his retirement he had been a painter and decorator for a local borough council; she worried unduly that at a recent outpatient consultation she had inaccurately described him as an 'interior decorator'. They were a harmonious couple, who never had any rows. Before the onset of her malaise they had enjoyed a full social life. They lived on their pensions and paid rent to a private landlord. The terrace is eventually to be demolished to make room for a council housing development, and they were both apprehensive about whether they could possibly find room for all their possessions in a modern flat.

Before her operation, or the symptoms leading up to it, Mrs Brown had been healthy. However, although never readmitted, she had continued to attend as a medical as well as a surgical outpatient at the great teaching hospital where the surgery had taken place, and had been treated by her GP with virtually the whole range of 'tricyclic' antidepressives and the minor tranquillisers.

At the interview she was noted to be unhappy, ill at ease and very anxious. Intellectually she appeared rather dull (though by no means subnormal) and kept turning to her husband to give information for her, which he did rather too readily. However, when pressed to answer for herself she could do so adequately, showing no confusion. Her hypochondriasis was to the fore, but was never delusional. She was physically fit, fully ambulant, and could see and hear normally. She was neatly dressed, though her untidy hair was in keeping with her generally flustered state. Her husband was much in evidence, large, kindly, composed and powerfully supportive.

The *formulation* was of a woman with a pretty normal background (for the East End) and previous personality, who had coped well with a fairly hard life during her first marriage, and retained the affections of her children. Her second marriage, to a middle-aged bachelor a few years her junior, had seemingly made few demands on her, and after the operation 10 years ago she had slipped into an increasingly dependent role. It seemed not unlikely that her husband colluded in this. For the past six years she had suffered bouts of depression of the milder sort, with prominent anxiety and hypochondriasis. Her identical twin also suffered 'nerves', so there might be a genetic factor. Apparently she had never shown anger in her adult life. The present bout, possibly a little worse than the previous one, might have been precipitated by her elder sister's death.

Treatment involved a social worker, whose task was to support Mrs Brown and her husband and help them be a little less dependent on each other. Social rehabilitation was attempted by introducing them both to a nearby pensioners' club; however, somehow the plan to loosen the tight marital partnership by Mrs Brown's attending a day centre fell through. A monoamine oxidase inhibitor (MAOI) was prescribed (an antidepressive of a kind which she had not received previously, more likely than the tricyclics to benefit this form of depression), and after two weeks she was considerably brighter and less anxious, though not wholly free from odd physical sensations. On this regime she remains relatively well, but as her illness has taken an episodic form it is too soon to say that she will not relapse.

Confusion and depression
Usually the *absence* of confusion is the most important distinction between depression and dementia. However, confusion and depression are found together: (1) where depression and dementia co-exist; (2) in depressive pseudodementia.

1. As dementia develops in one in ten of the senile population, and depression in perhaps one in four, it is hardly surprising that the two conditions should not infrequently occur together on the basis of chance alone. Also, to those who have insight into their progressive loss of memory and intellect, dementia is a dreadful affliction and actually causes depression. As has been described in the previous chapter, depression is especially common in the setting of *multi infarct dementia*, where personality tends to deteriorate much more slowly than intellect. While shallow emotionalism is commonplace in those brain-damaged by strokes, depression can be severe, especially where there is a family history of depressive illness. There may even be a constitutional connection between predispotition to severe depression and to atherosclerosis.

While there may gave been previous bouts of depression, at the time the patient with depression *and* dementia is seen it will be clear from the history that the dementia preceded this bout of depression. There will also be the other symptoms and signs of cerebrovascular disease (pp. 44–48).

2. Abstraction, retardation, and withdrawal in severe depression in the elderly sometimes impair orientation and the performance of intelligence tests; the patient may be too preoccupied with his mor-

bid thoughts to take in the questions, or too wretched to be bothered with them, or too slow to give the answers in the time allowed. Hence there is the picture of pseudodementia, to which the ageing effects of severe depression—the inactivity and slowness of the retarded depressive, the shakiness and irrational fears of the agitated, the bowed posture and shuffling gait—add colour. However, as explained on page 50, the 'dementia' is entirely due to the depression, and passes when the mood returns to normal.

Reactive depression

In my view this is not an illness at all, but a normal reaction to loss. Where the loss is very great, such as a sudden bereavement, or the discovery that one has cancer, the reactive depression is intense. Also, where the personality's tolerance of stress is low, the reaction may be extreme.

The main features of reactive depression are: (1) the depression is wholly justified by the subject's circumstances (as he sees them); (2) the mood varies with changes in these circumstances.

In young, immature or inadequate adults, reactive depression is often the basis of suicide attempts; in most cases the depression which gave rise to the attempt is rapidly relieved by the professional help and efforts at reparation by the nearest and dearest which usually follow admission to hospital. Though such behaviour is far less common in the aged, it does occur.

Mr White, 70, a bachelor living alone was admitted to a general hospital unconscious as a result of coal gas poisoning. On recovery he explained that he was awaiting an operation on his inner ear for a suspected cancer. In recent months he had seen a specialist at two different hospitals about the discharge from his ear. Twice he had been under the impression that all was well, and twice he had been sent for and told otherwise. Now the suspense of waiting for surgery, with a none certain result, and the prospect of pain and deformity had seemed too great, and he had attempted suicide. In hospital, however, with people to listen and take an interest and approach the surgeon on his behalf, he cheered up enormously. He had the operation, which was a success (at least, in the short term), and three months later was sent home. He was readmitted two days later, having made another suicide attempt, this time by taking an overdose of the antidepressive he had been given on his first admission, which had, unnecessarily, been continued during his stay, and of which he had, injudiciously, been given a supply on his discharge. Due to the overdose he was at first grossly confused. As a result of this and his grotesque appearance—he was wearing a woolly wig to hide the cleft where his ear had been and the operation had paralysed one side of his face—he was regarded by some of the staff as demented, and given a wide berth. However, within a day of his transfer to a psychiatric ward he was quite normal. He described how, on his discharge, he had felt frightened and desolate, and had suffered pain in the ear which made him fear a recurrence of the cancer. It was felt that he was suffering a purely reactive depression to the expectation of a lingering, painful death, and that while in company his spirits were easily sustained, in solitude his apprehension overwhelmed him. Consequently arrangements were made for him to go to an old people's home, where in due course he settled happily, there having been no signs of depression from the time of his recovery from the overdose.

While the stresses which provoke reactive depression are the same as those which often precipitate depressive illness, whether severe or milder in the elderly, the reaction in the former is much more immediate and proportionate to the degree of stress. In management, *relief* of the stress where ever possible, sympathetic *support*, psychotherapy to help the more stable and better preserved to come to terms with a situation which cannot be altered and short-term *sedation* over the period of acute crisis, all have a place, but there is little value (and, as illustrated in the case history above, possible harm) in giving antidepressive drugs.

The course of depressive illness
There is a natural tendency for depressive illness to get better. Even before modern treatments became available this was so, and melancholic patients in mental hospitals tended to recover spontaneously after a few months or a year or two provided they did not succumb to malnutrition, suicide or institutionalisation. Before the discovery of the antidepressive drugs, which made the detection of depression worthwhile, the milder mood disorders were not often diagnosed as such, but were more often labelled 'anaemia', 'fibrositis', 'vitamin deficiency', 'underactive thyroid', or 'the change'. Even so, in due course most remitted. Modern treatment makes less difference to depressive illness in the long than in the short term; the illness is cut short before it has run natural course.

Having happened once, however, depressive illness is extremely likely to recur. Relapse may be soon or not for many years. The pattern of subsequent episodes closely follows that of the first, with the same tendency to recovery.

Among the many ways of classifying depressive illness is that of recurring depression as *unipolar* or *bipolar*. The former means that the patient only gets depressed, the latter that he is sometimes manic too (see Ch. 8). Bipolar depression is far more likely to be helped by lithium therapy (see p. 84).

In old age, where environmental stresses are so important in bringing about depression, and the adaptability of the personality is diminished, the outlook for depressive illness is less favourable than in younger patients. Frequent relapses, incomplete recovery and chronic, intractable agitation and gloom are much more common.

Dr Felix Post of Bethlem Hospital (Post, 1962, 1972) showed that while treatment is successful in most patient in the first instance, there is subsequent invalidism—psychological and social—in about half of them. The following features are all associated with a favourable future—(and I am bound to say that few of them are typical in elderly depressives): age less than 70; a family history of manic or depressive illness; a previous history of severe depression (with full recovery) before the age of 50; an extrovert personality and an even temperament; severe, even bizarre symptoms, but a complete remission. On the other hand, a bad outcome is associated with older age and an aged appearance; evidence of brain damage, i.e. neurological signs or dementia; any serious, disabling bodily disease; and a history of uninterrupted depression for over two years. To these I would add, from my own clinical experience, chronic animosity, unacknowledged, between the patient and his or her partner, and collusion by a strongly supportive spouse or relative who unconsciously benefits from the patient remaining a dependent invalid.

The diagnosis of depressive illness

Except in hermits, severe depressive illness is very unlikely to be overlooked. Usually the depth of the depression, the vigorous self-denunciation, the marked slowing of speech and movements or the still more striking agitation, bizarre delusions of poverty or bodily disturbance, the typical sleep disorder and the variation of the mood through the day readily suggest the correct diagnosis, and correct hospital treatment is promptly arranged. Occasionally where hypochondriasis is especially prominent, admission is in the first instance to a medical or surgical ward for investigation of constipation or supposed inability to pass water, but the absence of physical abnormality and the patient's other manifestations of depression soon stop the pursuit of the red herring, and referral to a psychiatrist is swift. The diagnosis of depressive pseudodementia has already been thoroughly discussed (pages 50 and 73). The only other pitfall is where the histrionics of the agitated depressive lead the unwary to make a diagnosis of 'hysteria'. This term suggests both a particular kind of personality—shallow, emotional and attention-seeking—and a form of neurosis in which illness is unconsciously simulated for psychological gain. Often the distinction between these two meanings of 'hysteria' is not clear in the minds of those who use the word; in any case, both are highly misleading when applied to agitated depression. If the patient is regarded as a histrionic personality, her current distress may not be taken seriously; again, if she is suspected of 'putting it on', she may be denied sympathy and understanding.

Mrs Green suffered chronic agitated depression, which defied the best efforts of psychiatrists and other doctors in many different hospitals. She had many physical symptoms, which were energetically investigated. Minor abnormalities were discovered, such as osteoarthritis of her spine, for which she was given physiotherapy, a collar to wear round her neck and traction, with little benefit. Antidepressives and electroplexy were ineffective. She presented a challenge to every fresh doctor to whom she was referred, but she rewarded none by getting better. It was felt that the basic trouble was at home, where her passive, indulgent husband cosseted her, fostered her anxieties and failed to take with her the firm line which, increasingly, everyone else wished he would. Attempts to involve him in the therapy, however, were unproductive. Mrs Green was a 'pain in the neck'—a pain from which she suffered, and which she made others suffer too. She was relentlessly, boringly miserable, with a hopeless attitude to her future, continually seeking help but quite unable to use what was offered her. Psychotherapy was a failure—she was quite unable to express her feelings directly, or to see her difficulties in terms of relationships, but translated everything into her tedious 'body language'. She came to be regarded as a thoroughly inadequate personality, though there was little evidence that she had been so before she fell ill. She forfeited sympathy still further when she embarked on a series of flamboyant suicide gestures. She took two or three overdoses, but not under such circumstances that her life was really in danger. Twice on her way home she tried to throw herself from her husband's car. Twice she threw herself in the village pond; she came to no harm, though in fact the water was quite deep. Twice in hospital she threw herself down a flight of stairs, or said she had; X-ray after the second time showed a crush fracture of one of her vertebrae, so she probably was speaking the truth. However, all these attempts were felt to be tainted by 'acting out'. There was discussion about whether she should be relegated to a long-stay ward, or might be referred for a leucotomy. One night, however, she ended the controversy by going to the extremity of 'attention-seeking', and hanging herself from the curtain-rail around her bed in the ward. And the staff were left astonished and dismayed: 'We never thought she meant it.'

It cannot be stated too often that hysterical behaviour in the elderly must not be taken at face value, but is a manifestation of serious underlying disorder, much as fever is a sign of infection.

Milder depressive illness may be ignored, or misdiagnosed as a physical malady. The expectations of social behaviour in the elderly are so vague that an old person leading a very withdrawn and inactive life, staying at home and doing very little for months at a time, may not be regarded as abnormal. The decline into depressive apathy may be so gradual that the family and friends hardly notice what has happened, while those meeting the patient for the first time do not realise that is not the way he usually is. A survey in Edinburgh some years ago (Williamson et al, 1964) showed that general practitioners were unaware of three quarters of the cases of depression among the elderly at home. However, the community worker—social worker, health visitor, district nurse, home help, volunteer—who goes about her duties with 'wide-angle lenses', noticing what is happening to other people in the neighbourhood while attending to the client who is her immediate concern, is well placed to note when an old person has changed for the worse, by being more subdued, less responsive, less careful about appearances, or simply not being seen about so often. Enquiry may then elicit enough evidence of depressive illness to be drawn to the doctor's attention.

Both the apathetic and especially the hypochondriacal depressive may be regarded as physically ill. Thyroid underactivity, anaemia and Parkinsonism, for example, are conditions causing slowing and loss of energy for which depression may readily be mistaken, while the number of disorders sharing the symptoms of the anxious depressive is almost without limit: arthritis of the neck, restricting the blood supply to the base and the back of the brain, or pressing on nerves or the spinal cord; disease of the inner ear, causing giddiness; heart disease, causing shortness of breath or irregularities of the pulse (resembling palpitations) or chest pain; lung disease; peptic ulcer; disease of the liver, galbladder or kidneys; abnormalities of the bowel and womb; high blood pressure; diabetes; thyroid overactivity; arthritis; or cancer, anywhere.

Clearly, where the symptoms do suggest an important physical disorder, it must be excluded by careful examination and appropriate investigation. However, even if an abnormality is found, it may not be relevant to the patient's disability.

Mrs Black, 73, a widow living alone, had always been a rather neurotic woman, 'enjoying' minor ill-health, but leading a normally active life until she suffered a very small stroke, causing her briefly to pass out and lose her speech for a couple of days. Thereafter she lost the confidence to go out, and led a very restricted existence at home. A further blow was the move of her son, who had come to her daily from his work for the midday meal she provided, away from the district. She became miserable and lethargic and was referred to a general physician, who from her appearance, suspected thyroid underactivity. This was confirmed, beyond all doubt, by tests, and appropriate treatment was started. Soon there was no sign of hypothyroidism: her appearance, and the tests of thyroid function were normal. Her symptoms, however, were quite unchanged, and she continued to live a fearful, unhappy, inactive life. The physician referred her to the psychiatrist, who obtained the further history that Mrs Black had been previously treated for a depressive illness, 15 years ago, after the death of her husband; her symptoms then were essentially the same as now. She was treated with an antidepressive, induced to attend a day hospital twice a week (for company, stimulation, support and the 'reality testing' of her fears of sudden death or permanent disability) and within a month she was substantially better.

Mr Jones, a widower of 74, living alone, had heart disease causing irregularity of his pulse (but never heart failure), and had lost most of his vision as a result of a failure in the blood supply to the part of his brain registering sight six years ago. Though the pleasures of his life—reading, watching television, going round to the pub—were severely curtailed, he made a good adjustment to his disability at first. Over the past year, though, he had not been well; weary, anxious, troubled by pain in the upper abdomen, off his food, losing weight, unable to sleep without a sedative and even then waking early after only three or four hours. He was admitted to hospital for investigation just before Christmas with what he regarded as a heart attack—his heart had seemed very irregular, and he had been aware of alarming thumps and runs of beats in his chest. No abnormality was found which adequately explained all his symptoms. The possibility of cancer of the stomach was considered, but excluded by X-ray. The electrocardiogram though was abnormal, and treatment was given to regulate the beating of his heart. However, two days after his discharge he was readmitted, with palpitations and inability to cope. The psychiatrist then noted his glum expression and his inability to relax, sitting forward and constantly wringing his hands. When asked about his mood, Mr Jones readily spoke of the depression which made him wish to be dead, and the anxiety which rendered him fearful of dying. He said he had felt very lonely of late, and he viewed his future with great apprehension, but he agreed that loneliness did not entirely explain his depression. After three weeks on an antidepressive he was much more cheerful and confident, and was successfully discharged home with day hospital support.

In both these the history was strongly suggestive of depressive illness, and the physical findings distracted from the problem which mattered. As in dementia and as, indeed, in most of medicine, it is the history which makes the diagnosis. The history needs, however, to take account of the patient as a person, and not as a repository of potential diseases. Commonsense, linking effects with the most likely causes, rather than compressing or distorting patients on a Procrustes' bed of orthodox medical diagnosis, together with an awareness of the prevalence of depressive illness in the elderly, prevents error.

Milder depression can also be misdiagnosed as *reactive depression*, which matters if drastic measures are taken to modify the environment, e.g. rehousing, when what is needed is treatment for the depression.

Mrs Jacobs, long widowed, childless, in her 70s, living alone and more than content, usually, to be so, was sent into hospital by her GP suffering from acute loneliness. He felt that she needed an old people's home urgently, so urgently indeed that a place could not possibly be found for her soon enough, so he sent her to hospital for the time being. Attempts to discuss with her why, after so many years of being alone, she found the situation so intolerable were met with hostility and indignation: she wanted to be in a home, and that was that. It emerged that she had felt much like this for a spell in the wintertime yearly for some years, though never quite so intensely or urgently. Otherwise, however, she had no wish for company, shunned social gatherings, kept herself to herself and did not even bother to reply to the letters sent her by the surviving members of her family. Despite her protestations, a diagnosis of depressive illness was made, the loneliness being regarded as a symptom rather than a cause, and she was treated with an antidepressive. Over the course of three weeks her clamouring died down until she was readily persuaded to try a weekend at home. When she came back to the hospital she reported that she had felt quite happy, and asked for her discharge. All went well until the next winter, when she suffered an identical episode.

A *biochemical* test, the dexamethasone suppression test, which demonstrates the excessive production of cortisol by some severely depressed patients, can now be used to help diagnosis.

Treatment

Depressive illness should be treated quite as vigorously in the aged as in the young. *Severe* depression should nearly always be treated in a psychiatric ward; the patient who is extremely distressed, suicidal or taking too little nourishment needs observation and management of a skilled and tolerant staff.

Antidepressive drugs of the tricyclic and tetracyclic classes are of great value. The *tricyclics* are longest established, but tetracyclics may be preferred where there is a history of heart disease, notably irregularity, myocardial infarction or evidence of a conduction defect. The oldest tricyclic is imipramine (Tofranil), but it is probably best avoided in the elderly because it not infrequently causes alarming postural hypotension; when the patient gets up his blood pressure falls and he may faint. Amitryptyline (Tryptizol) has been available for about as long and is of more use to the elderly, who appear to tolerate its sedative effects rather better than do the young. Still more sedative is trimipramine (Surmontil) which can consequently be used for its hypnotic as well as its antidepressive effect. Sedation is useful for the agitated patient. Otherwise dothiepin (Prothiaden) is my first choice. It is generally effective and well tolerated. The most powerful tricyclic is clomipramine (Anafranil) but its anticholinergic side effects (which all tricyclics are liable to produce to some extent) are particularly marked: dryness of the mouth, sweating, constipation, sometimes blurring of near vision and retention of urine, and occasionally tremor too. The usual dose of all these drugs is 75 mg given once in the 24 hours, at night, though as little as 25 mg may suffice or as much as 150 or even 225 mg sometimes be required. For one drug at least, nortryptyline (Aventyl) there is a therapeutic 'window', and too much of the drug is as ineffective as too little. Consequently where it is possible to measure the level of the drug in the serum, the target is more readily and accurately reached.

Allied drugs, claimed to be as effective if not more so, safer for the cardiac patient and with fewer side effects are the *tetracyclics* mianserine (Bolvidon), nomifensine (Merital) and maprotiline (Ludiomil). These claims are probably best justified in the elderly by mianserine, which has few anticholinergic effects and is therefore better tolerated than some tricyclics and is safer for those liable to glaucoma and urinary retention. Whether it is ultimately quite as effective as some tricyclics has not been established, but it appears to act more quickly than the two to three weeks taken by those drugs. Sedation may however be a troublesome side effect. The dose is 30 to 60 mg at night. Maprotiline and nomifensine are both given in doses similar to those of the tricyclics. They are most often used as an alternative when tricyclics have failed, because they are relatively new and have not yet shown overwhelming advantages over other drugs. Theoretically, in view of the acetylcholine deficiency in the brains of sufferers from Alzheimer's dementia (p. 43), the less anticholinergic antidepressives are to be preferred in those depressives who are also confused.

Very agitated patients will also need a *tranquilliser*, usually chlorpromazine (Largactil). For those who are too drowsy on this, however, thioridazine (Melleril), or lorazepam (Ativan) can be given instead. Troublesome paranoid delusions are relieved by trifluoperazine (Stelazine) 10 to 20 mg daily; those on high dose, however, are likely to need a drug to prevent Parkinsonism, say orphenadrine (Disipal).

Nutrition must be observed carefully, and the daily intake and output of *fluid* charted wherever there is doubt that the patient is taking enough. The intake should not be less than 2 litres, nor the output less than 1 litre/day.

Where fluid intake is inadequate, the patient's anguish so great that the effects of an antidepressive drug cannot be awaited, where he is actively suicidal or where there has been no response to drugs, *electroplexy* (ECT) is the treatment of choice. The patient is rendered briefly unconscious by a short-acting anaesthetic, all the voluntary muscles of the body are thoroughly relaxed by an injection which follows the anaesthetic, and a fit is then induced by means of electrodes applied to the skull, which send a current of around 100 volts to the base of the brain for about half a second. It is not the electricity which is therapeutic, but the fit. The muscle relaxant to modifies the fit that the body merely twitches, but the brain is affected as if there had been a full convulsion. After a quarter or half an hour the patient is fully conscious, with no memory of the experience after the prick of the needle giving the anaesthetic in the first place, and now ready to continue the day's activities. Treatments are given twice a week (but more often at first if the patient is extremely depressed and not eating) to a total of between four and twelve.

ECT has had a bad press lately, mainly from those who are

neither psychiatrists nor severe depressives (Kendell, 1978) but withstands the attacks and remains an honoured treatment in psychogeriatric practice. We now have an idea about how it works, through its action on the biochemistry of the mid brain, though admittedly for many years it was an empirical treatment, i.e. it worked because it worked! The same used to be true of 'foxglove tea' for the failing heart, until eventually the action of digitalis was understood, and the same is still of true of the pain relieving effects of aspirin! It is not a way of frightening or 'magicking' the patient back into normality, though the effects are frequently dramatic. It is still, after 40 years, the most effective treatment we have for severe depression. Though the benefit is psychological, for the most part (though appetite, energy and sleep are also restored), the action is physiological, on the functioning of the brain. The treatment is remarkably safe (even for the very old), and modern techniques have rendered it a comfortable procedure which most patients take in their stride. The attitude to an elderly depressive of 'poor old thing—why don't they leave her alone?' is well-meaning, but totally misguided. Frequently ECT is a life saver, and it would be as negligent to withhold it as not to remove an obstruction from the windpipe of someone who was suffocating. Post (1978) in a farewell letter entitled *Then and Now* movingly describes the transformation of the plight of chronic depressives in the Crichton Royal Hospital following the introduction of electroplexy.

All patients, and the elderly more than most, may suffer a temporary loss of recent memory after two or three treatments. This always clears, usually in not more than six weeks, but may last longer and prove quite troublesome. The idea that this amnesia is what makes the patient better is quite wrong. It is a nuisance, and best prevented if possible, for example by giving treatments less frequently once the patient has started to improve, and by placing the electrodes over the side of the brain they use least, i.e. on the right side of the skull in a right hand-handed person.

It is objected that ECT is not a permanent cure, and that in due course the patient who responds is likely to relapse. This is true, as it is of all medical rather than surgical treatments. Successful cure of pneumonia by antibiotics is no guarentee that the patient will never suffer pneumonia again, but that is no argument for letting him die of it in the first place. Successful ECT cuts short *this* episode of depression, and to the depressive, living in a private hell, that is very worthwhile. It is in the nature of the illness that there is likely (though not certain) to be another episode, but not for months or years.

Often refusal of food and fluids responds to the first one or two electrical treatments, but if it does not, the patient's nutrition must be ensured by intravenous 5 per cent glucose or tube-feeding, until he will take enough by mouth.

Milder depression can usually be treated at home by the general practitioner, or at the outpatient clinic or day hospital by the psychiatrist. Again *antidepressive* drugs are very useful, and the *tricyclics* are the first choice. They are given as to severe depressives, but usually the lower doses set out on page 61 suffice. Side-effects are less well tolerated by milder depressives (who are not quite so distracted by their misery), so dothiepin (Prothiaden) is probably preferable to amitriptyline.

If however after a month the patient is no better, the alternatives of electroplexy or a *monoamine oxidase inhibiting antidepressive* (MAOI) must be considered. Electroplexy is indicated where the symptoms resemble those of severe depression 'writ small'; early morning waking and definitely feeling better at the end of the day are particularly good guides.

Electroplexy can quite safely be given to outpatients, provided they can be trusted to have eaten or drunk nothing for at least four hours beforehand, and there is someone to escort them home, as confusion may be marked for some hours after treatment. It can also be combined with antidepressive therapy of either type.

An MAOI is more likely to help the anxious, hypochondriacal depressive whose mood varies from day to day, who tends to feel worse at the end of the day, who has difficulty in falling asleep, and who is irritable as well as depressed. Though certain foods must be excluded from the diet—cheese, yeast extracts and pickled herrings—and other drugs must not be taken without a doctor's approval (see Ch. 15), MAOIs are very well tolerated by the elderly, and side-effects are very few. Phenelzine (Nardil) 15 mg three times a day is the most generally useful.

A few patients who do not respond to either class of antidepressive alone are greatly helped by both together. The combination is usually regarded as unsafe, but certain drugs in each class blend satisfactorily with each other. This is a specialised area of treatment, however, and should be practised by the seasoned psychiatrist.

Antidepressive therapy which has proved effective should be *maintained* with no reduction in dosage for at least three months. If the illness was of fairly recent onset the dosage may then be gradually reduced and discontinued over the course of the next two or three months. If the patient relapses, the original dose must be restored, and maintained for another three months before reduction. If there is again relapse, the drug had better be continued indefinitely. Likewise, if there is a long history of depression (i.e. a year or more) it is probably advisable not to stop the antidepressive. As yet we have no evidence that patients on long-term antidepressive therapy are at any risk from the drug, while they are probably at less risk from recurrence of the depression.

Alternative antidepressants include *flupenthixol* (Fluanxol) half to 1 mg twice a day, which sometimes bucks the patient up within a few days but is unlikely to help the severe depressive, and *lithium carbonate* (see next chapter) which rarely curtails the current episode of depression but may lengthen the gap between and the length of subsequent bouts.

Anxious milder depressives usually require one of the milder tranquillisers for a while, as well as an antidepressive. Chlordiazepoxide (Librium), diazepam (Valium) and oxazepam (Serenid) are about equally effective, Lorazepam (Ativan) rather more so, though some patients find it too sedative.

All depressives tend to sleep poorly until their mood has returned to normal, and may therefore require a sleeping draught or tablet for a spell.

The shorter acting *hypnotics*—chlormethiazole (Heminevrin), temazepam (Euhypnos, Normison), triazolam (Halcion) are appropriate where there is difficulty in falling asleep while the longer—nitrazepam (Mogadon), chloral hydrate, dichloralphenazone (Welldorm) are more useful for the classic depressive early morning waking. It is most important not to continue night sedation any longer than is necessary, and to this end the patient should be persuaded to start doing without it a week after there are signs that the depressive illness is remitting.

To complete the discussion of *physical* methods of treatment, a mention must be made of *psychosurgery*. There is a small, unfortunate minority of elderly depressives who make no worthwhile improvement on antidepressive drugs, alone or in combination, or to ECT. Their circumstances have been alleviated as far as is practicable, and every effort has been made to explore and expose states of conflict or unspoken hostility, but they remain wretchedly miserable. Some of these patients, especially those who are chronically tense and agitated, obtain striking and lasting relief by operations dividing the front(al) lobes of the brain from the thalmus in the mid-brain, thus severing the tracts which link thoughts with emotions. The effect is well expressed by the lay notion of 'cutting the worry nerve'. Formerly leucotomy (lobotomy), in which the fibres were cut with a scalpel, often caused undesirable personality changes, in the direction of selfish callousness, while admittedly relieving the tension, and the operation fell out of favour. In recent years, however, a greatly refined technique has been developed by Mr Geoffrey Knight, of the Brook Hospital in South London (Bridges, 1973). In the procedure of *sterotactic tractotomy* radioactive 'seeds' are very accurately placed, guided by X-rays, in the exact part of the brain where they will do most good and least harm, and the results has been most gratifying.

Most patients are substantially better, and very few indeed are worse. Those who do best include those whose lives have not been completely disrupted by depressive illness for too long. Anyone who has suffered agitated depression for 10 years will also have suffered prolonged institutionalisation, the effects of which the relief of tension alone can hardly be expected to undo. Patients should preferably be referred to the neurosurgeon when they have been continuously ill for less than two years, and before they have been virtually written off as 'hopeless cases'.

Psychological treatment begins with *empathy*, and the attempt to see the patient's depression as the outcome of a human problem. It is usually possible to do this without recourse to far-fetched speculations. 'Here and now' formulations, taking the personality, of course, into consideration, are of more value than theories based on the remote past, though serious loss at an early age is recognised as contributing to morbid depression following other losses in later life. Truly endogenous depression, unrelated to any apparent stress, is very rare in the elderly—rarer still when one considers that, as Sir Aubrey Lewis has commented (Lewis, 1934), the whole truth may not always be told, or the peculiar significance of certain seemingly ordinary events to the patient not be appreciated by the observer.

I am bound to confess, though, that in my experience, understanding of the 'dynamics' of depression, in terms of grief or frustrated anger, can rarely be shared with the patient in a way which actually relieves his distress. I have heard it claimed that severe agitated depression can be speedily dispelled by appropriate interpretation, but I have never seen it happen, and I have yet to be persuaded that the claim is anything more than a fantasy. However, insight into the patient's state of conflict within himself or with those about him is very helpful to those who try to treat him. They understand him as a person, and the sensitive areas which may profitably be explored during the period of treatment. They have clues as to why he behaves as he does and how he reacts to staff, and other patients. The phenomenon of *transference* explains how one sometimes treats those around one as if they were important people from one's past. Thus, for the patient the doctor may represent his father, the ward sister his mother, and the patients his brothers and sisters, rivals for parental love, transformed into powerful and effective treatment. The way he acts is both explained by and helps to explain his feelings about the key figures in his life. Perhaps most important of all, understanding the patient gives those treating him realistic expectations of what possibly can be achieved, and they do not waste time in the vain pursuit of trying to make silk purses out of sow's ears.

Mrs Thomas, in her middle 70s, had been depressed off and on for five years, since her husband, who had had an operation for cancer insisted on taking his discharge from hospital. During the next year, until his death, 'I never had a wink of sleep'. She insisted that they slept in separate rooms—'He wanted things which I couldn't mention to you'—which he resented. 'I had to lock the door. He said he wouldn't sleep in the back room, but it wasn't, it was my living room'. Until he died he was very difficult, but she denied that previously the marriage had been unhappy. 'Of course, he used to drink, and he'd had malaria, which made him violent sometimes, but we got on.' Since his death she had lived alone, often visiting her nine children, all married, none living more than a few miles away. 'They're very good children. They've got their own lives to live. I feel a burden to them. If I could live nearer to them I'd be all right'. She could not bring herself to say what was obvious from her manner, which was that she wanted far more of her children's company and resented their not visiting her, but when asked nodded briefly and went on to remark: 'They give me every material thing that I could want—but its not what I need'. She remained unable to sleep, which she attributed to the fear of break-ins, as she had suffered two minor burglaries in successive years. Before retiring she barricaded her front door with all furniture she could move, and she would get up very early and pace the landing in her dressing gown for hours. Several times in the course of the interview she exclaimed, 'If things don't get better I'll kill myself. I've nothing to live for really, have I?' Lately she had been so preoccupied by her misery that she had not noticed things, like who she met in the street; yet she was highly sensitive to what was going on round her, and worried that she was being commented on and gossiped about. 'Not that they'd have anything to say—I've always led a good life'.

She was a plump, well preserved woman, wrapped in a sleek fur coat. She told her story in an almost supplicating manner, with a

wealth of feeling, if not complete consistency. Her distress was evident enough; further, one soon had the feeling that one was being
made to take responsibility for it, and that her talk of suicide was
in fact a threat. It was easy to feel pressured, as perhaps her children were.

She leapt at the offer of treatment in a day hospital, but almost at
once said that she did not think she could eat the food provided
there—she was used to catering for herself at a very high standard.
When told that salads were often available she said that that would
be all right then, and went on: 'I dont't want you to think I'am
asking for any special treatment'. She ended the interview with 'I
hope I haven't been a trouble to you'.

Her story was shot through with rationalising, self-pity and denial—of the disgust she had felt for her dying husband, and her
anger at her children for leaving her so much alone. To put it
bluntly, she was a humbug. Recognition of this did not mean that
she was denied the treatment which her distress and the realities of
her plight warranted, but that the staff embarked on therapy with
their eyes wide open to the likelihood that she would be demanding, difficult to please and ready to play off one against another.
While there was no thought of completely exposing herself to herself, the plan was to help her talk more honestly about her griev
ances. It was also hoped, as she was one of the fitter and more
alert members of the day hospital, to deal with her dependency by
encouraging her to help the more infirm rather than being herself
so passive and helpless. Antidepressive therapy was prescribed; a
previous course of amitriptyline had failed, so phenelzine (MAOI)
was given instead, with reasonable confidence that she would feel
much more cheerful and relaxed in two or three weeks. It was fore-
seen though that while her mood should be brighter, her basically
insecure manipulative and highly defensive personality would remain. The best that could be achieved was to relieve her depression
and help her, though still neurotic, to function better.

Psychotherapy, which aims at increasing the patient's tolerance
and understanding of himself by frank discussion, has a place in
the treatment of depressive illness wherever incompletely acknowledged hostility seems to be a contributory factor, (but more often
as a complement to, than a substitute for, physical treatment). This
may need to involve other members of the family, especially the
spouse, in seperate interviews or jointly with the patient. The social
worker has an especially useful role to play here. In joint interviews
it is often possible for grievances to be expressed and considered
thoughtfully rather than reacted to in anger; the presence of the

professional 'third party' keeps the situation cool enough for the grounds for resentment to be examined objectively.

In the ward or day hospital *group therapy* frequently allows a freer airing of hostilities than is usually possible in the 'one to one' situation of individual psychotherapy. The discovery that one can actually criticise staff and fellow patients, and by doing so gain understanding rather than bring down retribution, may be therapeutic. Support by a group rather than a powerful individual person like a doctor, is less productive of dependency and regression (reverting to childlike behaviour). For some less tractable depressive illnesses, especially accompanied by regression and disturbed behaviour (e.g. screaming, collapsing, reluctance to leave bed, incontinence), *behaviour therapy* may achieve more than drug or hospital treatments or dynamic psychotherapy. The form most often used is *operant conditioning*, where the patient is consistently rewarded for desired behaviour, while the unwanted behaviour goes unrewarded. Suitable rewards for elderly adults are not all that easily devised, especially for depressives who take little pleasure in anything, but staff attention—a nurse spending a measured amount of time of exclusively with the patient, talking, listening or doing things with him—is often coveted in hospital, and choice items of food, sweets, cigarettes and outings may also be used. Ethical problems may arise in discouraging unwanted behaviour patients are not supposed to be punished like naughty children but it certainly must not be rewarded, and sometimes privileges are withheld, scant attention is given to extravagant 'sick demands' and the company of other patients likely to be distressed by childish and disruptive behaviour must temporarily be foregone. The help of a psychologist in setting goals and divising appropriate programmes to achieve them is invaluable.

Mr Warner, at 67, was only just in the psychogeriatric age group, but his depressive illness had developed very soon after his retirement 2 years ago, and he had never been mentally ill before. He was very severely agitated especially in the mornings, and was given to beating his head against the wall and threatening (but not attempting) suicide. He was married with five children all living away from home, and the marriage was under great strain; eventually it was discovered that his wife had taken to drink. Whether this strain was the cause or the consequence of his depression was never quite clear, but his wife and children were as keen as he that he should be in hospital.

Antidepressants and tranquillisers were of limited and transitory benefit. Attendance at a sheltered workshop and later at the Day

Hospital repeatedly broke down because of clamorous out of hours demands for hospital admission. After several months in hospital, during which courses of ECT, combined antidepressants, and intravenous clomipramine proved totally in effective, a sodium amytal abreaction (emotional release by the disinhibiting effect of the drug given, cautiously, intravenously) produced only more depression and his wife's cooperation in marital therapy proved elusive; psychosurgery was urged, but was refused. He seemed utterly stuck in hospital and destined to become a chronic patient there.

However, after the psychologist had found no evidence of dementia a behaviour modification programme was devised to discourage his histrionic 'helpless and hopeless' behaviour and foster independence. Very basic activities like getting up, dressing, washing, shaving, setting the table and fetching his breakfast were charted daily according to whether they were performed without help, with verbal prompting, some or total physical help. The staff's interest was aroused by implementing this programme, and their attention and approval were Mr Warner's main rewards. A not altogether expected bonus, however, was his wife's enthusiasm, participation and revival of some warmth towards him.

Within a fortnight his behaviour was much improved. He was doing everything for himself within the hospital, and while his mood remained rather lugubrious and defeatist, episodes of head banging became exceptional. He started to help some of his more disabled fellow patients, and was distracted from his gloomy self absorption while doing so. Before long he was spending days, then week ends at home. Not all of these were successful. Several times he was brought back sooner than had been planned by his distraught and exasperated wife. However, she learnt and practised the reward/discourage regime with the support and advice of the ward staff who frequently visited the home.

Three months after the programme had been started Mr Warner was discharged home, after almost a year in hospital. A community psychogeriatric nurse paid almost daily visits at first, to see that he did not slide back into his former regressed melancholy. He did not, but settled after a fashion, and attended the hospital five days a week to do woodwork, a former interest which he had regained.

He remained a withdrawn, nervous, uneasy man, subject to spells of frantic despondency but was capable of enjoyment at times, and no longer acted like a sick and fretful child. A lot of painstaking work had gone into his rehabilitation;—far more than in giving tablets or ECT-but for the time being it had worked.

The community nurse stopped visiting after some months because she was leaving. Mr Warner remained at home for another year, but the relationship with his wife deteriorated. They sought a place for him in a residential home and he has now been fairly settled in one without coming back into hospital for over three years.

Another technique is *assertion therapy*, based on the idea that depression is learned helplessness. The patient is encouraged to do anything he can, even to folding a table cloth or making a cup of tea, which will give him a sense of being less than totally incompetent. Then he makes a phone call, buys something from a shop, makes a choice about what to eat, and, in psychodrama or rôle play, sticks to a decision, has a point of view and even argues about it. Depression may dwindle as effectiveness increases.

Occupational therapy within the hospital (and at home in the few areas where the local authority provides it), the relief of relevant physical disabilities where possible and social rehabilitation—often by way of a day hospital, centre or club—are other important aids to the full treatment of depressive illness.

For those in whom the depression is a clear-cut illness in contrast to the normally functioning personality, treatment can finish soon after the symptoms have gone. For the majority, however, in whom the illness is less well-defined, where stress continues and recovery has been incomplete, on-going support is required, by continuing day care, attendance at an outpatient clinic, visits by a social worker or health visitor, or by the general practitioner. Any signs of relapse should be first met by recourse to those measures which originally proved most effective. It is discouraging when a patient with a well-documented history of depression responding to, say, tricyclic antidepressives or ECT relapses after two or three years and is then referred, with identical symptoms to those of the former breakdown, to a general physician for investigation of supposed anaemia.

Common sense is at a premium in the practice of psychogeriatrics but, unfortunately, not all that common.

REFERENCES

Barraclough B M 1971 Suicide in the elderly. Recent developments in psychogeriatrics. Brit J Psychiat, Special Publication no 6. Headley, Ashford
Bridges P K, Bartlett J R 1973 The work of a psychosurgical unit. Postgraduate Medical Journal 49: 855–9
Brown G W, Harris T 1978 Social origins of depression: a study of psychiatric disorders in women. Tavistock, London
Carney M W P, Roth M, Garside R F 1965 The diagnosis of depressive symptoms and prediction of ECT response. Brit J Psychiat 111: 659

Kendell R 1978 Electroconvulsive therapy. Journal of the Royal Society of Medicine 71: 319

Lewis A J 1934 Melancholia. A clinical survey of depressive states. J Ment Sci 80: 277

Lewis A J 1971 Endogenous and exogenous; a useful dichotomy. Psychol Med 1: 191

Post F 1962 The significance of affective symptoms in old age. Maudsley Monograph no 10. Oxford University Press

Post F 1972 The management and nature of depressive illness in late life. Brit J Psychiat 121: 393

Post F 1978 Then and now. Brit J Psychiat 133: 83

Seligman M E P 1975 Helplessness: on depression, development and death. Freeman, San Francisco

Williamson J, Stokoe I H, Gray S, Fish M, Smith A, McGhee Stephenson E 1964 Old people at home: the unreported needs. Lancet 1: 1117

Mania

Psychiatrists tend to fight shy of the word *mania* these days, and use the term *hypomania* instead. Hypomania means 'something less than mania', mania perhaps being regarded as a state so extreme that few ever attain it. However, we use the concept of depression to describe moods ranging from mild dejection to suicidal despair, and I see no reason why mania should not similarly delineate various degrees of pathological *exaltation*.

The manic patient is almost literally madly merry. He is full of fun, unless thwarted, when he can become surly, or even aggressive. He laughs and jokes and talks a great deal, as if under pressure. He quips and makes puns and rhymes. He is bursting with ideas, all of which he attempts to put into practice, simultaneously; but the day, though he gets up before dawn, and does to bed (if at all) well into the small hours, is not long enough. Despite his furious activity, his energies are misdirected, and little is achieved. He is hasty and slapdash; concentration is very poor, and persistence greatly modified. He craves company, and dominates any social gathering; at first the life and soul of the party, he soon becomes an overbearing bore. He is sexy, and much inclined, at the very least, to slap-and tickle. He spends freely and recklessly. He has no time to eat and sleep, but must forever be up and doing.

Though mania is the opposite to depression, the conditions are two sides of the same coin, bipolar depression. The manic's humour is truly sick. In a sense he laughs like the clown whose heart is breaking, so that he may not weep. Most of us from time to time practice 'manic denial', avoiding unpleasant realities by making light of them, using 'gallows humour', relishing black comedy, throwing ourselves into frantically energetic pursuits as a distraction from what is sad and disappointing. In mania it is as if this normal psychological defence is taken to a pathological extreme.

Every manic patient is also subject to bouts of severe depression, sometimes alternating with mania, sometimes more, sometimes less frequent than the manic spells. Thus the manic-depressive patient is either 'high', low or normal, though a few unfortunates spend almost the whole of their lives either manic or depressed.

The *constitutional* factor is of greater importance in mania than in pure depression. The great majority of manic patients have a family history of mania and/or depression. The personality classically predisposed to mania is extrovert, lively and jolly, very unlike the serious, obsessional person who is liable to depression only. Plump, Pickwickian people, short and stocky, with round heads on round bodies are more likely than those who are tall and thin to break down with manic illness.

While *precipitating* stresses are much the same as those which provoke depression, they are usually less prominent in mania, except when it occurs for the first time in old age. Shulman & Post (1980) found that elderly men who develop mania often have a past or recent history of brain injury, mainly due to trauma or to stroke.

Mania usually occurs first between the ages of 20 and 40. The onset may be sudden or more gradual, so that enough time may elapse between the patient's being thought to be in rare form, 'going like a bomb', and his recognition as mentally ill, for him to have brought himself to the brink of financial ruin, or other serious trouble. The usual *duration* of a bout of mania is around two months—time which passes very quickly for the patient, and very slowly for those who watch over him. After the first bout there may not be another for several years, but eventual relapse, or depression, on at least several, if not many more occasions, is virtually certain.

At all ages depression is far more common than mania. Manic illness accounts for no more than 1 in 20 admissions to the general psychogeriatric ward, while depression is responsible for almost half. Manic episodes in the elderly are often simply a continuation of a life-long tendency, but mania can occur for the very first time after the age of 65. Indeed, it does not show the tendency of unipolar depression to dwindle in the very old, and first ever admissions for mania actually increase with age.

Mrs Briggs, aged 79, was admitted to a psychogeriatric ward in a state of confused excitement six weeks after the death of her husband. There was no previous history of mental illness. The marriage had been a long and apparently happy one, but there were no children. A fortnight after the bereavement Mrs Briggs started rising very early and wandering her street half clothed. When the milkman called she ordered a pint for everyone in the road, confident that she could afford this gesture of goodwill. She became embarrassingly talkative, obtrusively friendly, and those who had expected to console her were nonplussed. As she was getting such a disappointing response from her neighbours, she turned her attentions to the police, pestering them at the station and repeatedly asking that a constable or two be sent along to keep her company. When they protested that they were short of officers, she stopped likely lads who were passing her home and urged them to join the Force. Her appearance was dishevelled, and she ate too little. Meals on Wheels were arranged, but she was rarely indoors to eat them. She was bland and frivolous about the way in which she was neglecting herself, and would not agree to go into hospital, but when eventually compelled she made no fuss—indeed, she treated the occasion as a huge joke.

In the ward she was found to be somewhat undernourished, but otherwise fit. She was rather fatuously jolly, and not truly confused; inattention at first caused her to seem so—she could not be bothered with the questions she was asked—but it was soon clear from her ability to retain what she was told, and the speed with which she found her bearings, that her memory was unimpaired. Her mood was not always elated; for half an hour at a time she would be quite sober and sensible, and able to talk about the loss of her husband in a wistful rather than a mournful way. Then she would become silly or flirtatious, boasting that she had thousands of pounds to spend (in fact she had nothing but her pension) and would live another thousand years.

She was treated for mild mania, and gradually her mood returned to normal. She was sent home, to continue with tranquillisers, and the full support of community services was arranged. Three months later she was readmitted with similar symptoms of mania, and since then there have been two more spells in hospital, one for mania and one for, at last, depression.

Mania in the elderly has certain special features:

1. *Confusion* at the outset, which may lead to a misdiagnosis of delirium. The more acute the mania, the more likely there are to be confusional features. These pass off after a few days, when the true nature of the underlying disorder becomes obvious. A previous history of manic or depressive bouts, and the absence of any signs of physical illness to account for delirium, help to make the distinction from the latter.

2. *Paranoia* is often prominent, to the point where the patient may be frankly deluded, hear hostile, hallucinatory voices and jollity gives way to peevish irritability. However, the liveliness and sociability of the paranoid manic are in marked contrast to the wariness and withdrawal of the paraphrenic.

3. *Depression* can occur at the same time, giving the intriguing picture of 'miserable mania'. This is rather like a jocular form of agitated depression—the patient is restless, unhappy and may indeed have depressive delusions, but expresses them waggishly, with rueful wit, unable to resist the typically manic 'flights of ideas' (where talk flows in a stream of casual associations) but with a morbid and melancholy content. Or there may be rapid switching from one extreme of mood to the other, so that the patient who is overbearingly hearty most of the day suffers brief moments of suicidal depression.

4. *Talkativeness* more often takes the form of being long-winded, and talking round the point (circumstantiality) than true flights of ideas. Consequently, the development of mania may not be recognised, and the patient be simply regarded as a very difficult person, and treated (or mistreated) accordingly.

Mrs. Davis had lived in old people's homes for two years. A sprightly old Welsh woman of 73, she had a reputation as a 'naughty' old lady who did not fit the compliant mould of the standard resident, and while some staff appreciated her as a colourful character, others resented her 'cheek', bad language and troublemaking. She had clearly had a troubled adolescence when she bore two illegitimate sons by different fathers, was labelled a 'moral defective' and sent to a large mental hospital in the North of England where she spent 15 years. After her discharge she cohabited for many years with a man who ill-used her. Her background was only sketchily documented, but it appeared that she was again in a mental hospital, this time in the South, before coming to London and obtaining a room, and a job in a pub. Surprisingly, perhaps, she did not drink, and kept going, apparently able to care for herself, until after her retirement. Then she got into difficulties with her rent, as she spent her money on trivia, neglected herself and fell out with her neighbours. After a lot of ill-feeling from those about her, aimed at the Housing and Social Services Department as well as the lady herself, a place was found for her in an old people's home. There she was found most difficult—noisy, rebellious and provocative—and on the strength of her past history a psychiatrist was asked to see her. He found no evidence of mental illness, though plenty to indicate personality disorder; she was still, it seemed, a disturbed adolescent, craving love and attention while needing to assert her independence and individuality by being outrageous, in the body of an old woman. His advice that 'what can't be cured must be endured' was not received gratefully, however, and as soon as a new home was opened in the borough she was among the first to be transferred there. She was furious, made a great uproar, wet the new carpet, tried to break out at night using her walking stick (she had an arthritic knee) against the glass of a locked door, generally making her presence felt. However, the matron was able to handle her with the firm kindliness she needed; soon they got on very well, and for the next year she settled down very happily.

Then, for no obvious reason, she again became extremely troublesome. Her temper flared more readily than before; she swore freely and once threw her dinner over an attendant. At night she would open her window and shout obscenites to passers-by. She protested vehemently that it was not she who made these scandalous outcries, but the old lady who shared her bedroom. However, when she was moved to a room on her own the shouts continued, and even induced some of those outside the home who heard her to make enquiries on her behalf. Her behaviour made little sense, because when confronted she had no lasting grievance, and insisted that she was very happy in the home and wanted to stay there. She talked and talked, from morning till halfway through the night, wearing her listeners out.

The general view was that this was Mrs Davis up to her tricks again, but the matron thought that there had been a definite change in her mental state, and arranged for the psychiatrist to call again. This time he felt justified in making a diagnosis of mild mania. Mrs Davis' garrulousness went well beyond what could be regarded as normal. She spoke at a great speed, not only about current events, but also about her past, bringing in reminiscences which had no apparent bearing on the present issues. She was taken away from the point not by rhymes, puns or other purely chance associations, but by her extreme long-windedness. She was at first distressed by the interview, pleading that she was not 'mental', did not want to be 'put away' again, and reminding the psychiatrist that at their previous meeting he had stated that she was not mentally ill. She was, indeed, completely alert, and said nothing deranged. She insisted that she was happy in the home, while admitting, disarmingly, that she was 'cheeky' now and then. She clung to her story that it was the other resident who had shouted those things at night, and promised that in future her conduct would be unimpeachable.

Her volubility, excitability, emotionalism and the story that she had become more disturbed lately for no clear cause all suggested a manic illness, and it seemed likely that this had contributed to what had been presumed to be manifestations of personality disorder in the past. She was treated with two tranquillisers—

chlorpromazine and haloperidol, and in a month had calmed down considerably, so that her happy relationship with the home was restored.

Treatment of manic illness is best undertaken in hospital. Even a mildly manic patient puts a considerable strain on his family and neighbourhood, and runs the risk of getting into debt or infringing the law. I recall one patient who started redecorating his house everytime he relapsed into mania, and had a different coloured wall to represent every episode of illness (as he never finished the job). Another would fill his home with pets which appealed to him—puppies, kittens, doves, chickens, tortoises—which his unfortunate wife had to dispose of whenever he was admitted to hospital. Another bought two expensive cars on the same day, with no driving licence and only £50 in the bank. And a fourth was sent to prison for writing an obscene letter to a teenage girl and stealing knickers from a woman's hostel—actions completely out of character. There is a still more serious risk, to life, in those who wear themselves out by extreme overactivity, taking neither rest nor nourishment.

The first obstacle to admission may be failure to recognise that the patient is ill, as illustrated by the examples recounted above. The second is the patient's lack of insight. As far as he is concerned, not only is he not ill, but he has never felt better in his life. A great deal of persuasion is needed, therefore, to get him into hospital, and not infrequently compulsory admission under the *Mental Health Act* is required (see Ch. 17).

In hospital (always a psychiatric ward) treatment is mainly with tranquillisers. Chlorpromazine (Largactil) and haloperidol (Seranace) are the most useful. Often they are best given together, when the disadvantages of oversedation by the chlorpromazine, and of muscular spasms from the haloperidol, may be reduced: a typical regime would be haloperidol 1.5 mg three or four times a day, chlorpromazine 50 mg three or four times a day and 100 mg at night. In the early stages, if the patient is unco-operative or exceedingly disturbed, either drug may be given by injection—chlorpromazine 100 mg or haloperidol 5 mg—up to three times a day. Orphenadrine (Disipal) should be given if haloperidol causes Parkinsonism (muscular stiffness, shaking and drooling), and extra sedation is likely to be required with the chlorpromazine at night—chloral hydrate, chlormethiazole or nitrazepam.

These drugs control, but only rarely abolish manic symptoms. The usual duration of a manic episode is 5 to 6 weeks, and this is not reduced, but the severity simply mitigated, by medication.

In recent years evidence has grown that a salt, *lithium carbonate*, is of value in the treatment of mania and in preventing or reducing the frequency of recurrences of manic-depressive episodes. Possibly the action is through effects on the metabolism of sodium, which lithium to some extent replaces. In the elderly the salt should be used if manic-depressive episodes are occurring more often than once a year, provided that there is no heart failure and the kidneys are working normally (otherwise there is a risk of toxic effects from an excessively high level of lithium in the blood). The usual dose is about 1 g a day, given as Camcolit, or the slow release preparations Priadel, Phasal or Liskonum. The dosage must be monitored by regular checks on the level of lithium in the blood, at first weekly, for one month, then monthly for six months, then every three months, to ensure that enough is being given to have a preventive effect, but not so much as to be toxic. Occasional side effects are a fine tremor of the hands, weight gain, and the passage of large quantities of water accompanied by thirst (nephrogenic diabetic insipidus). Early signs of lithium poisoning are shaking of the hands, muscle weakness, malaise, diarrhoea, nausea and vomiting, and if these appear the salt must be stopped and the blood lithium level checked immediately. Sometimes lithium therapy induces underactivity of the thyroid gland so a periodic check of thyroid function is advisable. The amount of sodium chloride (common salt) should not be restricted in patients on lithium therapy. Special care needs to be taken in those who are on diuretics. Not uncommonly patients who have suffered very frequent and regular relapses into mania or depression find that they are much reduced in duration and severity with much greater intervals of normality, if indeed they are not abolished altogether. If this is so, the benefits outweigh the disadvantages of any of the side effects mentioned above. Provided the patient is under careful supervision in the early stages lithium therapy may be started in out-patients. Tranquillising drugs may be needed in in-patients who are actually manic as well as lithium until the mania has subsided.

Before the introduction of chlorpromazine in the early 1950s, severe mania was treated by electropley, as many as three treatments being given in a single day until the condition came under control. Now the only use of ECT is for mixed depression. In less severe cases 'miserable mania' responds to combined tranquilliser and antidepressive, e.g. haloperidol and amitriptyline.

The staff caring for the manic patient must be patient, persuasive and, when the occasion demands, firm. As so often in psychogeriatrics, a sense of humour helps a lot, too. Their task is to contain the patient, see that he takes his tablets, and gets enough rest and nourishment without feeling intolerably restricted. Physical restraint is rarely needed: seclusion in a side-room is harsh unless the patient is so overactive as to require heavy sedation for a day or two, and a locked ward is unnecessary. The patient should be up and about, mixing with his fellows and as fully occupied as possible, with a wide range of activities (to none of which he will apply himself for very long) including physical exercise; the occupational therapist has an especially important part to play here. Until he can be relied upon not to run off, the patient is best kept in dressing gown and slippers—an effective and unobtrusive form of mild restraint.

In my experience a manic patient is often a tonic to a psychogeriatric ward. While he may irritate other patients, they also identify with his outrageousness and disrespect, and it is therapeutic for them to find that, however awful he is, the staff do not reject or suppress him, and that under their ministration he makes a full recovery.

REFERENCES

Shulman K, Post F 1980 Bipolar effective disorder in old age. Brit J Psychiat 136: 26

9

Paranoid states

Morbid suspicion is a feature of most psychogeriatric disorders.

Paranoia on the basis of *confusion*, in delirium and dementia, has already been described (Ch. 5 and 6). In *delirium*, where the patient is anxious and perplexed, forgetful and unable to think clearly, and liable to misinterpret his environment by seeing or hearing things as other than they are, paranoia develops very easily. For a short while he feels trapped, imprisoned, persecuted, the victim of unthinkable horrors, and he reacts with panic and aggression. However, the delusions are poorly formed and fleeting; there is a distraction, or a sudden change of mood, and for the time being the paranoia is past.

A paranoid phase, often lasting several months, is common in *dementia*, usually in somewhat domineering personalities. The awful implications of a failing memory are denied, and instead the mental mechanism of projection is used to blame others: 'Everyone keeps muddling me up and taking my things'. Paranoid ideas are of this degree only, and never develop into the organised delusions of paraphrenia (see below), but the attitude can be one of sustained grievance, causing much unhappiness to the family and thorough disruption in an old people's home. With the progressive intellectual deterioration of dementia the paranoia eventually passes, but until then it responds disappointingly to drug treatment. For example, trifluoperazine (Stelazine), so useful in the treatment of most paranoid states, is more likely to be physically disabling than to relieve the paranoia in the presence of confusion.

Paranoia in association with *affective illness* has also been described in Chapters 7 and 8. It is a feature of *severe depression*, when it may be frankly delusional. However, while the patient is distressed to feel looked at and talked about critically, he is more likely to feel that this hostility is justified than to resent it. In *mania*, paranoia may be directed towards those who try to curb the patient's enthusiasm, or be rationalised by the supposed jealousy of those who do not share his imagined gifts and good fortune. While he treats this jealousy with enjoyment or disdain, the reaction to restrictions regarded as wilful and arbitrary is occasionally violent, if short-lived.

Paranoid *personalities* (see Ch. 11) are those who go through life with 'a chip on their shoulder'. They are either extremely sensitive and oppressed by feelings of inferiority, deeply wounded by slights, real or imagined, and nursing grudges, or aggressive and belligerent, picking quarrels and ready to go to law at the least pretext. They are an especial problem in old age, either because with ageing they have become 'more like themselves', and are thus more difficult and cantankerous than ever, or because their attitude to others over the years has alienated those who might help them and left them isolated and at increased risk from the hazards of ageing, or because in a dependent position (such as requiring the services of a home help, or being admitted to hospital, or residing in an old people's home) they are found intolerably fractious and demanding. The paranoid personality is well illustrated by the case history on pages 122–123.

Conditions *predisposing* to paranoia include:

1. *Sensory deprivation*, especially *deafness*. Inability to hear readily leads to misinterpretation of what is said, and a paranoid construction can be put on perfectly innocent remarks. Deafness is frequently exasperating both to the sufferer and those who try to communicate with him, and perhaps this sense of annoyance feeds the paranoia. Indeed, many deaf old people are virtually cut off from social contact by their deafness—most people find the effort of trying to talk to them too great—and their isolation contributes to the paranoid process. The moral is to obtain a hearing aid early in the course of deafness, before social breakdown, because afterwards the patient is unfortunately most unlikely to learn how to use one effectively.

Blindness, though to a lesser extent, also conduces to paranoia. The acute deprivation of sight which follows some eye operations, though only temporary until the bandages are removed, is sometimes associated with a transitory paranoid reaction.

In fact any major procedure in hospital which leaves the patient apprehensive, uncomfortable, baffled, unable to move much and uninformed may precipitate an episode of acute paranoia. This includes major surgery such as the replacement of a valve in the heart, and the sometimes strange and alarming experience of being in intensive care.

2. *Exhaustion*, such as may follow a serious illness or operation, or accompanying chronic debilitating disorders like bronchitis or

severe arthritis, seems to evoke paranoia. The model of 'brain-washing', where the victim is uneasy, uncertain and sleepless may unwittingly be reflected by the pattern of existence for some such patients in institutional care. The peevish invalid, who feels neglected or discriminated against, occasionally becomes frankly paranoid. Probably the more patients are treated like adults, the more personal care they receive, the better their amenities and, above all, the better communications are within the institution, so that staff really know what they are about and the patient is kept fully in the picture, the lower the level of paranoia.

3. A *foreign* environment: *immigrants*, trying to adjust to a strange country, culture and language are particularly susceptible to paranoia, ranging from the very common fears of prejudice and victimisation to florid illness. For many patients, of course, a hospital is a foreign environment, as can be an old people's home to the elderly.

4. *Illiteracy* is conducive to paranoia. Not only is the illiterate old person handicapped by being unable to read or write and liable like those who are deaf or foreign to misinterpret information, but also there is often a sense of shame at being so ignorant which heightens sensitivity to supposed slights and criticisms.

5. *Drugs* used in the treatment of physical illness occasionally provoke paranoid reactions, for example the steroids (like cortisone) and some of those used against tuberculosis and Parkinsonism.

Certain of the drugs of *addiction* are also associated with paranoia in various ways. Excessive quantities of the amphetamines (e.g. Dexedrine, Methedrine, 'purple hearts') cause an acute paranoid state which resembles one form of schizophrenia, but lasts little longer than the excess of the drug in the body. (Amphetamine addiction, however, is virtually unknown in the elderly.) The withdrawal of barbiturates from those who have become dependent on a regular high dose sometimes precipitates a brief episode of paranoia. Chronic alcoholism is associated more often than can be explained on the basis of chance alone with the development of a chronic paranoid illness very like (some would say, indistinguishable from) the paranoid form of schizophrenia.

6. Certain *physical diseases* affecting the functioning of the brain but without necessarily causing either delirium or dementia can cause paranoia. For instance, one of the various forms of 'myxoedematous madness' (Asher, 1949), due to thyroid underactivity, is paranoid, and there is a tendency for severe epileptics to develop a serious paranoid disorder after 15 years or so of their illness.

PARAPHRENIA

The most distinctive and well-defined of the paranoid states in the elderly is *paraphrenia*. Here the paranoia is not simply due to an attitude, an exaggerated response to stress, a colouring of confusion, or a disturbance of mood, nor is it related to any obvious physical cause, but it is the principal feature of a mental illness in its own right.

The paraphrenic patient is typically *female, solitary, partially deaf* and *eccentric*, but without a past history of serious psychiatric illness (Kay & Roth, 1961). In later life, usually past the age of 65, she starts to build up extraordinary *suspicions* of her neighbours. She believes that they talk about her critically. At first she may deduce this simply from their gestures, which she believes refer to her; if she sees them conversing, she feels they must be talking about her. Later she actually hears *hallucinatory voices*, which are loud, rude, very real to her and consequently disturbing. Sometimes the voices are confined to one or two rooms, usually the bedroom and the bathroom or lavatory, where they comment on what she is doing in a hostile, belittling manner, or abuse her directly. Sometimes she hears them all over the house, but she can get away from them by going out. Sometimes, however, they pursue her wherever she goes.

She believes that she is spied upon with telescopes or television cameras, with wireless and microphones and tape recorders; that noxious gases are blown in under the door, strange lights shone through the ceiling (though visual hallucinations are rarely prominent), that powder is sprinkled on her food, the water poisoned, that she is attacked with radiation, and that her electricity is stolen. These *delusions* are usually strictly *localised* to the people next door, upstairs or across the way, and are not attributed to the whole neighbourhood or the world in general. They do not fluctuate from day to day but are strongly sustained.

A common belief is that there is a mysterious machine in the locale, used for a nefarious purpose and making a noise, night and day, which no-one else can hear but which keeps her awake. *Erotic* delusions are not unknown—'That man down the road is trying to seduce me with X-rays'. One patient of mine, a 70-year-old spinster and never mentally ill before, believed that she had been raped, nightly, by remote control and that she had conceived a brood of tiny babies which lived inside her and fed off the interior of her breasts. Another variant on the persecutory theme is the belief that somewhere nearby and within earshot a child is being ill-treated, usually by its cruel parents. The paranoia is then on behalf of this unfortunate little one rather than for the patient herself.

The *response* to these delusions and hallucinations is generally quite appropriate. Some patients are frightened and move away, if they can—but if they manage to do so the persecution almost always starts up again in the new neighbourhood within a matter of months. Others complain to the police, and are sufficiently reassured that the matter will be looked into; I suspect, indeed, that the police may be better informed than any other agency about the incidence of paraphrenia in the community. The more aggressive abuse their supposed persecutors roundly, or even attack them physically, and thus themselves become objects of complaint. Others go into a state of siege, behind doors with half a dozen locks and as many bolts, sometimes insulating their walls against harmful influences by elaborately arranged sheets and blankets. In such a situation there is an obvious danger of self-neglect. Very occasionally paraphrenic patients feel so oppressed that they attempt suicide.

The intellect is quite unimpaired, and confusion is never a consequence of paraphrenia. A few patients use private words (neologisms), or ordinary words in a private sense (metonyms) to describe what their persecutors are up to, but otherwise can converse quite normally. Unless they go into a state of siege, they usually look after themselves quite adequately.

Post (1979) describes three forms of paraphrenia:

1. The patient's delusions are strictly localised to one particular neighbour who is heard talking sometimes to her and is believed to enter the patient's dwellings and interferes with her belongings.

2. A schizophreniform type where delusions are more widespread often extending into the neighbourhood and the street. There are ideas of reference so that people seen talking together are thought to be talking about the patient, car lights are flashed ominously, special optical devices and bugging are used to spy on the patient and there may too be jealous delusions about the spouse.

3. A schizophrenic type, almost identical with paranoid schizophrenia in younger patients, in which the subject hears herself discussed in the third person, experiences passivity feelings, e.g. being influenced from a distance or having her thoughts read. These are characteristic features of schizophrenia, though a family history of that illness so prominent as a rule in younger schizophrenics is usually lacking. Personality tends to be better preserved and thought disorder is confined to occasional neologisms and metonyms as described above. These differences and the more

appropriate emotional and behavioural responses are explicable by the paraphrenic's more established and mature personality at the age when the disease develops.

Paraphrenia occurs in perhaps 1 per cent of the population over 65 and accounts for a little more than 5 per cent of patients over that age admitted to the psychiatric wards.

Untreated, paraphrenia runs a chronic, unremitting course, and once fully developed is likely to continue unchanged until the patient's death. As she has no insight at all into the fact that she is ill, she is unlikely to seek medical aid except to relieve sleeplessness and general distress secondary to the feeling of persecution, unless the doctor is seen as a powerful potential ally. Never the less, paraphrenia is less likely than other psychiatric disorders to go unnoticed probably because its effects are so often troublesomely obtrusive. Rehousing is often sought and sometimes helps, but usually only transitorily.

It is fruitless to argue with the patient about her delusions. Often without agreeing whole-heartedly, one goes along with them, or at best, agrees to differ. Treatment may be rationalised as a means of fortifying the patient against her harrassment (see below).

In milder cases, where the patient can be relied upon to take the tablets prescribed, treatment can be given at home. A day hospital may be suitable for a few. But most require admission to a psychiatric ward for a spell. Some may accept this readily, being grateful for a refuge from their persecutors; others require a great deal of persuasion, and not a few will only come in if compelled to do so by an order made under the *Mental Health Act.* Such an action is justifiable if the patient can be regarded as a danger to others (which is very unusual) or to herself (by self-neglect) or so greatly disturbed and distressed as to need treatment urgently (see Ch. 17).

Once admitted, many patients leave their hallucinations behind them, though not their delusions. The response to phenothiazine tranquillisers, such as thioridazine (Melleril) or trifluoperazine (Stelazine) in adequate dosage, is usually excellent. Within two or three weeks hallucinations are abolished and delusions no longer troublesome. Insight, however, is rarely obtained. The patient does not say 'I was ill' or 'I imagined it' but 'they've stopped it!'

Unfortunately, compliance with medication is especially hard to ensure in the paraphrenic patient who often feels that it is not she who requires treatment but her persecutors. This problem may to some extent be overcome by 'salesmanship'. Without arguing about the persecution one may be able to persuade the patient that she needs to fortify herself against it by getting sufficient rest, which the tablets or capsules will provide. Occasionally an agreement may be reached that the doctor recognises the remote possibility that there could be substance in the patient's beliefs but thinks they are far more likely to be due to mental illness.

A trial of medication will then perhaps clarify who is right! Sometimes it is wise for the psychiatrist to ask his more trusted and better known GP colleague to prescribe. Persuading the patient to attend a day hospital or enlisting the aid of a community psychiatric nurse also helps to improve compliance.

Even so, many patients who have been persuaded to start treatment give it up after a while. At first they may feel better for doing so—anti-Parkinsonian drugs may not completely abolish the phenothiazines' tendency to produce muscle stiffness—and when the voices return a few weeks later they fail to see the connection with having stopped treatment.

To overcome this common difficulty, there are long-acting phenothiazine preparations, *fluphenazine decanoate* (Modecate) and *flupenthizol decanoate* (Depixol) which, given by intramuscular injections last for from one to several weeks. They are as effective as Stelazine given daily by mouth over the same period, and are of great value in keeping the paraphrenic patient untroubled by her delusions. The injections can be given on the occasion of the domiciliary visit, at the doctor's surgery, the outpatient clinic (many psychiatric departments run special clinics for the purpose), day hospital, or by the visiting community or district nurse. The chief drawbacks of these drugs are their side effects, the same as those of Stelazine: tremor, stiffness, unsteadiness, restlessness and drooling. Also, the injection once given cannot be withdrawn. It was disconcerting to discover that the commonest single iatrogenic cause of admissions to a joint geriatric/psychogeriatric unit was the use of depot-phenothiazine injections! It is therefore the best policy to treat paraphrenia only when the condition is truly troublesome. Use the lowest dose of the phenothiazine least likely to produce side effects, be especially cautious in the presence of confusion or physical infirmity, use oral medication when compliance is at all likely, and be alert for signs of Parkinsonism so that anti-Parkinsonian drugs may then be given. It is probably better not to give anti-Parkinsonian drugs routinely however, as the risk of the later development of tardive dyskinesia (troublesome involuntary movements developing long after the commencement of treatment and usually irreversible) may be thereby increased. For these reasons thioridazine (Melleril) up to 300 mg daily should probably be tried first. If that fails trifluoperazine (Stelazine) should be given in a dosage from 10 to 45 mg per day (given as 5 mg tablets or 10–15 mg 'spansules' which release the drug gradually into the body over the course of 24 hours). If an injection proves necessary it is wise to start with a test dose of 6·25 mg Modecate or 10 mg Depixol and observe the effects over the next two weeks before deciding how much to give subsequently. Most patients are maintained on 25 mg Modecate or 20 mg Depixol monthly. Most *will* need to have an anti-Parkinsonian drug as well and unfortunately there is as yet no long-acting preparation of any of these, so one must rely on tablets, say orphenadrine (Disipal) 50–100 mg three times a day being taken by mouth: happily, it seems that patients are more prepared to do this than take a phenothiazine.

Close follow-up is essential if relapse or seriously disabling side effects are to be prevented. There is something to be said for an occasional 'drug holiday' in patients who appear to have responded very well to medication to determine whether the treatment is still necessary.

Post (1966) found that of 71 paraphrenic patients treated with oral phenothiazines 14 (20 per cent) recovered fully, 29 (41 per cent) recovered fully without full insight, 22 (31 per cent) made social recoveries only, retaining some abnormal ideas, and only 6 (8 per cent) made no improvement at all.

The prognosis over an average follow-up period of three years was closely related to the maintenance of drug therapy. Three quarters of those making a complete remission remained well, but it was possible to stop the drugs lastingly in only seven patients.

Occasionally a treated paraphrenic becomes classically depressed instead.

Miss Isaacs, a Jewish spinster of Russian origin, aged 69 and living alone, had had several admissions to a psychiatric hospital in the last six years, usually as a compulsory patient, for paraphrenia. She believed that her landlord wanted to evict her, and put large rats into her flat to frighten her. The neighbours gossiped scandalously, accusing her of promiscuity and self-abuse, and they kept her awake with a machine which made a whirring sound all night, on which they were cooking chickens whose feathers filtered down through the ceiling into her hall. She would be admitted after a furious row with these neighbours, often involving the police, and at first she would be sullen, hostile, and bad-tempered. In hospital, however, she always settled down on Stelazine and became a droll, quite good-humoured lady. At the time of her discharge, about a month later, she would be on good terms with the staff though she never acknowledged that her admission had been justified. She would return to her flat still believing that her landlord and the neighbours had been against her, but that they had now been warned off. She would continue to take the Stelazine under outpatient supervision for three or four months, then stop it, default on her outpatient attendances, relapse into her delusional state and in due course be readmitted as before.

On one occasion, though, when she became ill a month or so after stopping Stelazine she presented a different picture. She complained that she was very ill, and staggered about the room to prove her point. She was particularly bothered about her bowels which, she said, had virtually stopped, and consequently she was afraid to eat. She felt very weak, and it was too much effort to go out, clean the house or even change her clothes. She never slept well, but now, worse than ever. She wanted help, but it was an ordeal to ask for it. Any superfluous questions were resented, and enquiries about her past paranoia were dismissed: 'Don't talk nonsense!' She readily accepted admission to hospital where, after physical examination and investigations to exclude a cancer or other serious disease of her bowel, a diagnosis of depression was made. There were no features of paraphrenia beyond continuing lack of insight into her old delusions. She made an excellent response to ECT and was discharged on combined antidepressive and phenothiazine therapy. At the time of writing (nine months later) there had been no relapse.

One might postulate that the internal psychological conflicts projected in the paraphrenic illness are resolved otherwise when that outlet is blocked by drug treatment, and the result is sometimes depression. On the other hand, it may simply be that the phenothiazine causes depression as an occasional side-effect.

Footnote
It may have occurred to the thoughtful reader that the diagnosis of paranoia is open to abuse. 'I'm nobody's fool, you're suspicious, he's paranoid'. To describe a person as paranoid simply indicates an attitude, and is no more an indication of mental illness than is to call someone conscientious or slovenly. However, such a label can have dire consequences for the elderly, whose theoretical rights are often infringed on the grounds of expediency. For example, if the matron of an old people's home does not get on with one of the residents in her charge, or an old lady obstinately refuses to budge from her home when the council wishes to proceed with slum clearance, or where a private landlord wishes to be rid of an unprofit-

able tenant, the fear and resentment which the old person quite naturally feels under stress may be labelled paranoia and pressure put on the health or welfare services to take action on the grounds of mental illness. Consequently all allegations of paranoia need to be examined critically, and all the circumstances carefully examined, before the conclusion is reached that the 'patient's, attitude is unjustified, and that there is a psychiatric disorder.

REFERENCES

Asher R 1949 Myxoedematous madness. Brit Med J 2: 555
Kay D W K, Roth M 1961 Environmental and hereditary factors in the schizophrenias of old age ('late paraphrenia') and their bearing on the general problem of causation in schizophrenia. J Ment Sci 107: 649
Post F 1966 Persistent persecutory states in the elderly. Pergamon, London
Post F 1979 The functional psychoses. In: Isaacs A D, Post F (eds) Studies in geriatric psychiatry. Wiley, Chichester

10

Neurosis

Neurosis means much the same as the lay term 'nerves': a tendency to get overwrought. Neurosis is sometimes contrasted with *psychosis*, the latter designating a severe mental illness involving a loss of contact with reality and liable to require treatment in hospital, while the former is considerably milder, leading to a distortion of but no detachment from reality, and is normally treated, if at all, at home. As the joke has it, the psychotic says 'Two and two make five'; the neurotic, 'Two and two make four—and I can't stand it!'

Traditionally psychiatry recognises three forms of neurosis; the *anxiety state*, in which there is excessive anxiety, free-floating or related to hypochondria or specific phobias; *hysteria*, in which the anxiety is eased by 'conversion' into physical disability or loss of memory for whatever seems to be the focus of anxiety; and *obsessional compulsive states*, in which the anxiety is displaced by recurrent unpleasant or irrational thoughts, or warded off by tiresome rituals.

In old age, neurosis appears to occupy a narrow and ill-defined territory between the milder forms of depressive illness on the one hand, and personality disorder on the other. The diagnosis is made far less often than in younger patients; is this because neurosis is actually less common, or because doctors get used to their ageing neurotics, and do not notice the onset of neurosis in old age?

In the Newcastle survey already quoted (Kay, Beamish & Roth, 1964), however, there was a prevalence rate among elderly subjects living at home of depressive and neurotic states of 26 per cent. These were identified by the presence of one or more of the following symptoms: spells of depression, anxiety, tension or irritability; phobias or panic attacks; anxious hypochondriacal preoccupations; bodily disturbances suggestive of the physical symptoms of anxiety (e.g. palpitations); hysteria, or the hysterical exaggeration of physical symptoms. These are, indeed, the main manifestations of neurosis in old age.

While that study did not state how many of the 26 per cent were judged neurotic and how many depressed, a later report by another Newcastle worker, Klaus Bergmann (1979), gives more detailed information. He found that where the condition has developed after the age of 65, approximately two-thirds of the cases were diagnosed as depression and one-third anxiety state. Where the disorder had been present for some years before 65, and was merely continuing into old age, approximately half were suffering from anxiety state, one-third from depression and the remainder from personality disorder. There were roughly equal numbers of patients in the late onset (i.e. after 65) and chronic (i.e. developing before 65) groups.

Depression has been dealt with in Chapter 7, and personality disorder will be described in Chapter 11. The only true neurosis in Bergmann's study is *anxiety state*, which seems from his findings and those of his colleagues to be present in about 9 per cent of the elderly. This is not much below the figure for the prevalence of neurosis in earlier adult life, so the diagnosis is probably made so infrequently because, like milder depression, anxiety states in old people are often overlooked: 61 per cent were unknown to their general practitioners in the survey by Williamson et al (1964).

Anxiety, like depression is a normal emotion. *Healthy* anxiety has an obvious, immediate cause: a stress requiring a 'girding of the loins' for action, either 'fight', if the challenge is one that can be met, or 'flight' if it cannot. Muscles tense, ready for strenuous use; the heart beats faster, to increase the blood supply to those parts of the body which are to be exerted, the rate of breathing increases; the bowel and the bladder are emptied; sweat breaks out, to cool the body which will be heated by action and the mind is alert and active, concentrating on the task in hand. Thus we are prepared, by the action of adrenaline and autonomic (automatic) nervous system, to make a special effort in an examination, an important interview, a race, or to escape a charging bull.

Morbid anxiety has no adequate cause in the patient's eyes, though the basis may be fairly evident to others. The anxiety has, at first, no focus or object, but pervades mental life, acting as a handicap rather than a stimulant. The patient is restless, fidgety and cannot relax. His concentration is impaired, and as he does not take things in, he cannot recall them. He is irritable, and intolerant of noise. He lacks appetite, and has difficulty in getting to sleep.

Such a state does not usually last for long. Very soon a cause is found by the patient for his anxiety in physical ill-health. The physical manifestations of anxiety become the basis and justification of his fear. Muscle tension can produce aching or odd sensations almost anywhere in the body; palpitations suggest heart disease—the commonest fear; overbreathing suggests shortness of breath and can cause unpleasant dizziness and tingling in the hands and feet; the overactive bowel implies cancer, and the frequent passing of water, diabetes or kidney disease; sweating means fever; and the inefficient memory of the anxious preoccupied mind augurs cerebral tumour or madness. Now there is something definite to worry about, but the greater the worry, the worse the symptom, so a vicious circle is set up.

Another means of focussing anxiety is by developing a fear of special situations, or *phobia*. The anxiety mounts to the point of panic in these situations, which tend, therefore, to be avoided. Here anxiety and avoidance set up another vicious circle, which tends to perpetuate the phobia. The situations most commonly feared are those of travelling, crowded shops, or even of leaving home at all.

In the elderly, frank phobic states are uncommon and the common form is the anxiety state linked to the fear of ill-health. These may, however, be the rationalisation of a fear of leaving home, akin to agaraphobia in younger people, i.e. a relatively small physical disorder causes disproportionate disability.

Ironically, *actual* ill-health is the commonest *precipitant* of neurosis in old age, and seems to be of more significance than social stress. Neurotic old people have more often had a poor relationship with their parents and spouse than the normal elderly, and thus perhaps are predisposed to a neurotic reaction when they become ill.

Mrs Jarvis, a widow of 73 living with her single daughter, a full-time secretary, was admitted to a psychogeriatric assessment unit with a story of falling. She had been in medical wards on three occasions in the past two years, and on the first occasion had been found to have suffered a small, recent coronary thrombosis. The subsequent two admissions had been for faintness and palpitations, but on neither occasion was any further evidence found of physical disease. Prior to her referral to the assessment unit she had been in a state of great anxiety, ostensibly about her heart, fearing that it would suddenly stop, but actually about being on her own by day. To reassure her, her daughter had a telephone installed, but rather regretted having done so when her mother called her at work two or three times a day; indeed, her exasperation as much as any fears the doctor had about the old lady's health contributed to the admission.

She was the youngest of seven children, and apparently rather spoilt by her father, and felt that her mother disapproved; anyhow, she had never been as close to her as to him. She married, after working in shops, at 20, and was left by her husband 19 years later, with three children. Her brothers and sisters rallied round, however, and she raised the children without herself having to go out to work. The elder two got married, while the younger daughter did not, and stayed with her. They had been moved to a new flat six months before Mrs Jarvis developed the chest pains which led to the diagnosis of coronary thrombosis.

In the assessment unit she was not observed to have any palpitations, and there was no new evidence of any cardiac or other bodily disease. She was quite cheerful, and one of the ward's livelier patients. However, she described an episode of faintness when walking to the hospital shop, and another when she was on her own in the lavatory.

From the history rather than any positive findings a diagnosis of anxiety state was made. It was apparent that she had become very dependent on her daughter, especially since moving from the familiarity of her old home, and that anxiety symptoms were focussed on her heart by the episode of coronary thrombosis. While there was no previous history of psychiatric disorder, she seemed always to have been a somewhat nervous and immature person.

This formulation was discussed with her, and she eagerly accepted the offer of appropriate help: diazepam (Valium) 2 mg three times a day, and attendance at a day centre while her daughter was at work. The daughter was given the opportunity to air her own anxieties, guilt and resentment before the social worker; she disclosed that for the past 18 months she had been seeing a regular boyfriend—a married man separated from his wife—which, she felt had unsettled her mother, though she had no intention of marrying him.

This management has proved effective. Mrs Jarvis enjoys the day centre, and no longer needs the Valium. Her daughter sees the social worker from time to time, and the old lady has kept out of hospital now for almost a year.

This case well illustrates the most common genesis of anxiety state in the elderly. An episode of physical illness (especially affecting the heart) heightens feelings of insecurity already present because of the personality and the circumstances. Insecurity leads to anxiety, which causes bodily symptoms resembling those of physical disease, which increase the anxiety. The patient then flies for security, to the doctor and the hospital. Reassurance that there is 'nothing wrong' is then inadequate—the problem of insecurity must also be met.

Cardiac neurosis, an anxious over-reaction to heart disease, is, perhaps, the commonest form of anxiety state in the elderly. As was obvious from the furore which followed the first cardiac transplant, the heart means more to most people than merely an organ which pumps blood through the body, but is the centre of 'being'. Thus any threat to the heart is seen by many as a threat to their very existence, and if they are already insecure, the response is excessive.

Morbid thoughts and feelings are very common after myocardial infarction (coronary thrombosis) and make a substantial contribution to chronic disability after the event.

The term *hysteria*, when properly applied, refers not to mere emotionalism, nor to a particular kind of show-off, attention-seeking personality, but to a specific neurosis which takes two forms, each of which has the effect of relieving an anxiety state at the cost of physical or mental function. *Dissociative* hysteria, in which the patient forgets what it would be disquieting to remember, and has therefore a gap in his memory, though his ability to recall what he has just been told is unimpaired, is unknown in the elderly. The other form, in which anxiety is somewhat mysteriously *converted* into a physical symptom which gets the patient out of having to face up to an intolerable stress, such as 'I couldn't bear to see my daughter get married, and now that I'm blind I can't' is very rare. It only occurs, in fact, in that very small minority who have habitually, since adolescence, used this means of defending themselves against painful realities. When hysteria develops for the first time in old age it always indicates a serious underlying disorder, such as severe depression (p. 18) or a cerebral tumour, to which the patient is seeking, by desperate and primitive means, to call attention. However, the *hysterical exaggeration* of disability due to physical disease is by no means unusual in dependent personalities who are afraid to face the difficulties of life alone. This may delay or prevent full recovery from a catastrophe like a stroke: the patient may be afraid to get better (like a wounded soldier afraid of being returned to front line) in case he should be alone and stranded should the disaster recur.

Obsessional-compulsive states rarely arise in old age, but sometimes having begun in earlier life are especially troublesome in later years. An *obsession* is a recurrent, unwanted, irrational and persistent thought. A *compulsion* is a repeated action, based upon an obsession, which must be performed or the patient's tension becomes intolerable, e.g. hand-washing arising from an obsession with contamination by dirt, or checking again and again to ensure that the gas has been turned off and the front door locked. It seems likely that both obsessions and compulsions are means of controlling anxiety which come readily to obsessional, tightly controlled personalities.

Miss Blyth, a spinster schoolteacher of 70, had spent 21 months of the last two years in a mental hospital because of a crippling obsession that she would snatch babies from their prams and kill them. Her fear of doing this was so great that she did not dare leave her home except to seek refuge in a hospital ward. She had first had this trouble, to a much lesser degree, at the age of 50. It passed off after a few months, but returned from time to time, causing her great distress. Since her retirement at 60, when she found herself a comfortable maisonette in a busy street of a well-to-do London suburb, the obsession had bothered her far more often and more severely. Although she liked her home she frequently regretted living in so populous an area where she could hardly go out without meeting a pram. Her life became more and more limited. She would only go out to shop in the early morning, or after dark, and then ultimately not at all.

No treatment had given her worthwhile relief—neither physical, with various tranquillisers, and antidepressives and ECT, nor psychotherapy, aimed at bringing to full consciousness the jealousy and aggression which the obsession seemed to symbolise. Yet her intellect was quite unimpaired and her personality, though somewhat rigid and narrow-minded, was well preserved. In view of her lack of progress and the severity of her disability, she was referred for psychosurgery, and a stereotactic tractotomy (see p. 84) performed. The result was immediate and lasting. Her obsessions dwindled till they were mere unpleasant notions which in no way frightened or impeded her. She was able to return home and at last enjoy her retirement, leading a normally active life and becoming a keen member of a music appreciation group.

TREATMENT OF THE NEUROSES

This is essentially a blend of symptomatic therapy with social manipulation, support, psychotherapy and behaviour therapy as has already been outlined in the section on the treatment of depressive illness in Chapter 7.

The patient with anxiety state and fears for his physical health must first be allowed to give a full account of his symptoms, without being cut short and handed a prescription or sent away for investigations. Next there should be a careful enquiry into the present circumstances of his life. Often at this stage the cause of the anxiety will become apparent; sometimes, just as he is telling his story, the connection between how feels and what is happening will become clear also to the patient, who is thus enabled to understand his symptoms and see them in perspective. Next the past history is obtained, to show what kind of a person this is, what sort of family he came from, how he was brought up, how he coped with work and retirement, marriage and parenthood, bereavements and other special stresses, and which illnesses he has experienced. The picture, however, is incomplete without a physical examination. It is necessary to make quite sure that there is no serious or relevant physical disease, and the patient may rightly question any reassurance that he is physically fit unless he has been examined. If the findings at this stage are negative, though, further investigations should be kept to a minimum. Anxious patients find plenty to worry them in the mystique of hospitals and X-ray departments, and the more they are looked at by different doctors, all of whom give a slightly different impression, and the longer the delay before being told that there is 'nothing wrong', the less effective reassurance is likely to be. 'Doctors won't tell you everything' or 'My case was a complete mystery to them' or 'There must have been something wrong, or they wouldn't have put me through so many tests', are frequent comments indicating that the clean bill of health is looked at askance.

It is, of course, never sufficient to say 'there's nothing wrong with you'. The patient knows he had symptoms, and if told there is nothing wrong will conclude either that the doctor is a fool or thinks him a fraud. Reassurance must be reinforced by explanation of how anxiety can produce physical symptoms and why this may be happening at this time. The logic of prescribing pills or capsules which relieve anxiety will then be seen, and the patient will not feel fobbed off. Depending on the duration of the symptoms, the personality and the circumstances, further management may take the form of regular support (by an individual or a group, in a club or day centre or hospital), or psychotherapy, to increase self-knowledge and deal more healthily with the problems giving rise to the anxiety, which may involve the spouse and other members of the family as well as the patient.

Mr Gordon, 79, living with his rather younger wife and their unmarried son, suffered from a chronic anxiety state mainly focused on his stomach. He had had part of his stomach removed for a duodenal ulcer 11 years ago, and had not reallly been well since. His bouts of abdominal pain and vomiting had led to several more admissions under the surgeon after the first operation, and his abdomen had been opened up three or four times so that they could see if there was anything wrong; usually there was not. He was a thoroughly miserable-looking old man, deeply boring on the subject of his insides, and so deaf that it was very hard to talk to him. He was managed as a day patient which eased the tensions with his wife, who found his symptoms hard to tolerate, and gave him a measure of security in that he was always 'under' a hospital even though it was for 'nerves.' However, in the course of a year there had been four referrals to the surgeons and one more 'look-see' operation (laparotomy).

One morning I was asked to see him because his wife reported that he had been in a bad way all night and needed admission. However, the old man did not confirm this, and seemed indeed no worse than usual. Having a little time to spare, and feeling in good voice, I asked him to tell me about himself. To my surprise, he was most interesting. He told me of his tough childhood, of the warring East End gangs, of his political activity with the Labour party, and about the General Strike of 1926. He told me of how strong and fit he had been, and of his pride in his craftsmanship as a bricklayer. He showed a shrewd appreciation of the current political situation, and his ideas were clearly his own. Every time he wandered on to the subject of his symptoms, I gently steered him back on to the far more rewarding subject of himsef. Three-quarters of an hour slipped by very quickly, and I treated him with new respect.

A few weeks later I went to see him at home, and we had another interesting chat. He was an intelligent man, poorly educated but self-taught, and quite widely read. His wife listened to our conversation in amazement 'I don't know what's got into him,' she exclaimed, 'he never talks like that.' Poor Mr Gordon never got the chance: she was in no way his intellectual equal, and had come to regard him as a decrepit invalid, to whom she owed a duty but for whom she provided little love. Instead, her son had come to take over many aspects of his role, and father was pushed aside. This situation (almost an enactment of the classical Oedipus triangle, and by no means unique in psychogeriatric practice), together with his loss of substance and vigiour following the gastrectomy, seemed to be the basis of Mr Gordon's chronic anxiety.

He is not cured, but ever since then it has been possible to distract him from his symptoms by paying some attention to himself whenever the pains have been especially troublesome, and in 18 months he has not been back to the surgeons once.

Learning to *relax* is a helpful aid to the control of anxiety, and one which gives the patient a welcome sense of self mastery. Breathing exercises, classes, records, tapes, or a form of mild hypnosis can all be used to this end. Yoga and transcendental meditation develop the techniques to a fine art, and there is no reason why tense old people should not be encouraged to use them.

The *drugs* of most use to relieve *anxiety* are the 'minor' tranquillisers of the *benzodiazepine* group—which include chlordiazepoxide (Librium), oxazepam (Serenid), diazepam (Valium), medazepam (Nobrium), clobazam (Frisium), and lorazepam (Ativan), all of which have a calming effect on the mind through their action on the brain, while diazepam in particular also relaxes tense muscles. Diazepam is the most widely used, lorazepam probably the most powerful. There is some danger of dependency on these drugs but there is none to life if an overdose is taken; whereas the barbiturates, equally effective sedatives, were much more likely to induce dependency and quite often fatal if taken in excess. Propanolol, a beta blocker, relaxes the body without calming the mind, is neither sedative nor habit forming, and is often useful.

Sleeping tablets should be used with care, and prescribed, where necessary, in courses of no more than a month at a time, rather than indefinitely. Habituation develops all too easily, and an old person who relies on sleeping pills year in and year out may suffer withdrawal symptoms, such as confusion, if they are inadvertently withdrawn, or on the other hand may accidentally take an overdose. Again, a benzodiazepine, such as triazolam (Halcion), temazepam (Normison, Euhypnos) or nitrazepam (Mogadon), or alternatively the chloral-derived dichloralphenazone (Welldorm) or chlormethiazole (Heminevrin), are preferable to barbiturates.

Depression is a common accompaniment of anxiety states, when an *antidepressive* may be useful as well as a tranquilliser. The treatment then is essentially similar to that of the milder depressive illnesses (see Ch. 7).

The most important point in the treatment of *hysteria* is to recognise that there is an underlying problem to be identified and dealt with. Purely symptomatic treatment is as inappropriate for hysteria as it is for delirium. Because some symptoms appear to be 'put on' it does not follow that all are, and alertness to the possibility of physical disease or severe depression presenting in an unusual way is vital. The great danger of the diagnosis of hysteria is that it may close the mind to subsequent developments. Where the basis appears to be purely psychological—a hysteria-prone personality in conflict with her environment—they attempt to resolve the conflict by exploring and discussing it with all the parties concerned, 'having things out' where this is likely to help, and easing pressure by manipulation of the environment where possible, are of more value than challenging the patient's symptoms and trying to remove them by demonstrating inconsistencies, or suggestion. She should, however, be encouraged to expect improvement in any disabling symptoms in due course. The therapeutic team need to be consistent and unanimous in their approach, for hysterical patients are apt to 'divide and conquer', even if this means cutting off their nose to spite their face.

Where problems are chronic and virtually insoluble, regular *support* may reduce the need for symptoms, i.e. the patient 'seeks attention', so that is just what she is given, usually as a reward for refraining from clamorous demands and disruptive behaviour.

Support also has an important place in the treatment of *obsessive-compulsive* states which, in old age, are generally especially chronic and intractable. A more probing form of psychotherapy is rarely effective and may even aggravate symptoms. Obsessional personalities are usually too flexible to look at themselves from the outside, and have great difficulty in seeing the wood for the trees.

The course of obsessive-compulsive states is usually a series of worse spells with relatively untroubled periods in between. Often the worsening seems to be related to depression, and the use of an antidepressive may give relief. Otherwise tranquillisers of the benzodiazepine group, used in the treatment of anxiety state, are of most value. Behaviour therapy may relieve the intensity and urgency of compulsive behaviour, and, by thought stopping, (e.g. thinking of something very nice as a welcome distraction from the painful obsession) of obsessive thoughts.

Chronic and severely disabling obsessive-compulsive states in the elderly should not be allowed to continue for more than a year or two when the above treatments (with the addition of ECT where depression is especially prominent) are of no avail without recourse to psychosurgery. The stereotactic tractotomy is very well tolerated by such patients, and the results are frequently as gratifying as in the case of Miss Blyth (p. 115).

Doses of drugs referred to in this chapter are given in Chapter 14.

REFERENCES

Kay D, Beamish P, Roth 1964 Old age mental disorders in Newcastle-upon-Tyne. Brit J Psychiat 110: 146
Bergmann K 1979 Neurosis and personality disorder in old age. In: Isaacs A D, Post F (eds) Studies in geriatric psychiatry. Wiley, Chichester
Williamson J, Stokoe I H, Gray S, Fish M, Smity A, McGhee A, Stephenson E 1964 Old people at home: their unreported needs. Lancet 1: 1117

11

Personality and behaviour disorder

Delinquency, at its peak in adolescence and early adulthood, falls off with ageing, and the crime rate for the elderly is very low. Similarly the diagnosis of *psychopathic personality*, which is based on a record of impulsive aggression and irresponsibility, intolerance of frustration and inability to learn from bitter experience, is hardly ever made in old age. Presumably as they age some psychopaths mature and become more stable, some die of addiction or suicide, some, perhaps, express their antisocial drives vicariously, through their delinquent children, some become hypochondriacs and few 'old lags' remain in prison.

The increasing introversion which is a part of psychological ageing has a mellowing effect on the psychopath's ferocious extroversion. On the other hand, where the personality was always introverted—reserved, retiring and inclined to brood—such traits are exaggerated by ageing, sometimes to a troublesome degree.

Personality disorder is not a form of mental illness, though frequently referred to the psychiatrist. The 'disorder' is the failure of this particular person to fit into his present environment harmoniously. The complaint may come from the 'patient', unhappy to feel a misfit, or more often, from those who have to live with him. The problem is essentially a social one. Usually those difficult, eccentric, querulous, morose, miserly, unhygienic or disinhibited old people who get referred to a psychiatrist were ever thus, if not always to the same extent. In the past, however, they were fairly free to be themselves, to go their own way, and those who did not like them could avoid them. Most, consequently, are quite isolated in later life. However, increasing infirmity in old age forces them into a situation of dependency and hence potential friction with others.

The term *behaviour disorder* is borrowed from child psychiatry, and refers to certain forms of antisocial conduct, such as incontinence, living in filth and sexual misbehaviour, which do not obviously arise from any mental illness and are not readily understood as manifestations of the previous personality either. However, the dividing line between personality and behaviour disorder is not all that clear, the management of the two conditions is much the same, and in this chapter they will be considered together.

Withdrawal is a not uncommon cause of anxiety to neighbours and community workers, when an old person at home leads the life of a recluse, and seems at risk from self-neglect or ignores normal standards of hygiene till there is felt to be a possible danger to the public health. Only about half of these cases are explicable by mental illness–depression, schizophrenia, paraphrenia, or dementia. The remainder seem to choose this way of life for reasons which they can rarely explain. One such old lady was admitted to hospital having collapsed in a state of semi-starvation. She explained that it had been more and more difficult for her to reach either the front door or her kitchen. The reason was very clear when a visit was paid to her home; over the years she had accumulated so much junk, apparently throwing nothing away, that her flat was completely filled with it. The rooms were crammed to the ceilings with rubbish, the bath was buried beneath it, the hall and passages were so cluttered that one had to fight one's way through refuse, and the door to the kitchen was completely blocked. Yet in hospital she seemed mentally quite normal. An even weirder, more selective instance of *hoarding* was an elderly couple who spent every penny they had on cigarettes and matches, till their home was stacked like a tobacconist's shop. The kitchen contained little food, but was piled high with unopened packets of cigarettes, while between their twin beds was a block of a gross or so of matchboxes. The anxiety expressed by their neighbours was of the fire hazard. The couple explained simply that they were smokers.

Dr Duncan Macmillan (Macmillan & Shaw, 1966) coined the phrase *senile squalor syndrome* for those old people he found in his survey in Nottingham who seemed actively to reject society's standards of cleanliness, and lived in their own filth. Typically the persoanlity was domineering, quarrelsome and independent, and offers of help were resisted. When compulsion was used to force the patient (or offender) into institutional care while the home was cleared up, there was an almost invariable relapse into the former squalid state within months of the return home. Sometimes the condition is known as the Diogenes syndrome, after the famous unwashed cynic who eventually lived in a large earthenware jar.

Miserliness may be mentioned here. Very occasionally an elderly eccentric starves himself in order to save his meagre income. The money is usually not entrusted to a bank, but kept in a vase or stuffed into the mattress on which the patient may eventually be found, ill with malnutrition.

Difficult old people are just as common as difficult young people. Clashes take place particularly when they are in care—in a long-stay ward, or, most often, an old people's home.

The *paranoid* personality has already been described (p. 101). An example of the problems such a person may encounter because of his aggrieved attitude is afforded by the case of Mr Shooter.

He was a nice-looking old countryman of 80, with watery blue eyes, a thick thatch of grey hair, a weathered complexion and a hoarse voice. He had worked as a farm labourer, and was never an easy employee, but was mainly occupied in solitary tasks, worked well and got by socially despite his grumpy disposition. He never married, and after his parents' death was looked after by his elder sister till she died, leaving him alone at 76. He was unable to fend for himself in his tumbledown country cottage, and protested vehemently to the social worker who visited him. She was able to find him a flatlet among 30 such for old people, under the supervision of a resident warden, in a town five miles from his old home. From the moment he moved in there was trouble. Nothing suited him, and it was everyone else's fault. He still could not fend for himself, though he was physically and intellectually capable of doing so. He was supplied with Meals on Wheels, but complained consistently about their quality, always wanted what was not available, and refused to pay. When they were stopped in consequence he was more outraged than ever. He fell out with his home help within a fortnight. Nothing she did was right: 'she was lazy, dishonest, a loose woman and spread gossip about him'. Not surprisingly, after a month she refused to attend him any more. He fell out with his neighbours, accusing them of being noisy and ignoring him. He was a perfect pest to the warden, demanding her attention at all hours by means of a bell which was connected to her flat, and wearing her out with grievances till she felt she could not call her soul her own. When she was not available he would sometimes go out and 'collapse' in the street; when taken to his doctor or the local casualty department, however, he would not complain of any illness, but of neglect an unfairness.

Three months after he went to the flat he was transferred to an old people's home, where he was thoroughly disgruntled and disagreeable from the outset. He did not like the single room he was given, and he did not like the company in the double room with a better view he was offered as an alternative. He thought it wrong that he could not have the use of his full pension while in the home, and no amount of explanation would satisfy him that part was properly withheld as a charge on his keep. He quarrelled with the other residents, and said that they shunned him. He could agree with no one when watching the television—it was too loud, too soft, or the wrong programme. He made a great fuss over meals— they were too hot, cold or unsuitable for him, but protested that he was starved if he did without. He even told passers-by, 'They're starving me in there', and begged for money or a crust of bread. He aroused their indignation on his behalf, which did nothing for the morale of the harrassed staff. Repeatedly he threatened to leave, and occasionally he did so, but he never got very far before 'collapsing' as he used to before entering the Home.

The psychiatrist who was asked to see him sympathised with the staff's difficulties, but explained that Mr Shooter's paranoid personality was no form of mental illness, but the kind of old blighter Mr Shooter was, and that medical treatment could not help. Yet he prescribed a small dose of a tranquilliser, not because he thought that Mr Shooter would be made more bearable thereby but in the hope that the staff, under the impression that something was being done, would tolerate him better. This hope was in vain, for the old man resolutely refused to take any tablets at all: 'You're not poisoning me!' He was transferred into another home, and another, and another, before being slipped one weekend into the mental hospital of the psychiatrist who had seen him. The psychiatrist was not well pleased, and stated emphatically to the local authority that this was a misuse of a psychiatric bed, and that it was the authority's duty to find a suitable niche for Mr Shooter and staff who would put up with him. However, his protests fell on deaf ears, and Mr Shooter remains in the hospital on this day (three years later). Actually, he has been much less trouble there than anywhere else. The staff, being well used to awkward patients, do not take his complaints to heart, and treat him with good humour. Though the amenities are below the standard he experienced in the homes he was in, he enjoys a fairly free, independent life, and though he never expresses any satisfaction, he appears as contented as so prickly a personality is ever likely to be.

Stubborness can be exasperating or, in ill old people at home, dangerous (see p. 15). Those who are set in their ways may not change them even when it is essential to do so to survive. Some obstinately cling to their independence when they are well past being able to manage for themselves, and suffer in consequence or even die. An old man with gangrene of the foot refused adamantly to go into hospital though assured that unless he had appropriate treatment the trouble would progress, and he would die. An old lady with diabetes refused to cooperate with her insulin injections, and would not agree to admission even when there were clear signs that she was on the brink of a diabetic coma. Both died.

Extreme *dependency* is a major problem in those who anticipate a lonely, unloved old age in which they will be infirm or suddenly taken ill and have no one to care for them. Often after an unhappy insecure childhood they have functioned reasonably well as adults, with the role of their occupation, spouse, or parent to play, but as they get older they feel that they lack purpose and worth and are liable to be set aside, rejected and forgotten. They therefore constantly solicit care, usually on the strength (or weakness!) of imagined or exaggerated physical complaints or threats of suicide, and as almost inevitably their overtly manipulative demands alienate those whose help they seek, their plight becomes ever more desperate. One such lady called out the ambulance so often that when the crew discovered who had made the call they would exclaim 'Oh not you again!' and turn round and leave her. Almost every weekend she would seek hospital admission via her nearest casualty department, and her noisy misbehaviour in the middle of the night more than once led her fellow tenants to petition for her removal from their midst! Such people are liable to manoeuvre themselves prematurely into old people's homes, where they tend to lead fretful lives among very disabled demented and infirm residents ten or fifteen years their senior. It is far better if they can be found a function which increases or restores their sense of worth, for example, as a staff helper looking after less able older people in a day centre or hospital.

Less serious, but still trying, are those set *habits* which cause friction. For instance, I once met an extraordinary little old woman in an old people's home who crooned to herself and sang her every remark in a high nasal whine. The lady who sat next to her told me, with tears in her eyes, how insufferable she found this weird noise, day in and day out. 'I can understand that', I remarked, 'but why do you go on sitting next to her?' 'Why' the old lady replied, 'this is *my* seat.'

Disinhibition is displayed by a small proportion of the elderly, who exploit their venerable status by tactless and unduly frank remarks which cause consternation in families, and great embarrassment and resentment in homes. 'La vieille terrible' revels in her outspokenness, while she makes others squirm.

A more serious, and rarer form of disinhibition leads to *sexual misbehaviour* in old men. This is not, as is generally supposed, the first sign of dementia, but a more complex disturbance occurring in those with a past history, not of sexual offences but of impotency problems. The objects of the misbehaviour are children, for whom an old man's grandfatherly qualities have an appeal, whereas young women will not respond to him sexually. Exhibitionism and mutual genital fondling are the chief expressions of sexuality; more serious assaults are fortunately very uncommon. While public concern for the child in such an encounter may be entirely proper, the consequences for the old man are frequently tragic.

Mr Graham, a 90-year-old widower, lived alone in a terraced house at the bottom of a back-street in a working-class London suburb. He was visited by one of his three children every weekend, and during the week was seen to by a home help who lived in the same street and had known him all her life. A psychiatric consultation was sought because it was rumoured that he had interfered with little girls in the park. The police reported two or three incidents when he was thought to have his hand up a child's knickers, or her hand inside his flies, though charges were never preferred.

He found to be a delightful old man, short and round as a ball, with a large walrus moustache through which he smoked his beloved pipe. He was a little deaf, but alert and, apart from his obesity, very fit for his years. His home was as compact and cosy as a gnome's. It seemed improper to broach the sordid subject of the consultation, which was therefore approached in a roundabout, gingerly way. He gave not the slightest indication that there was any substance in the allegations which, when at last they were brought into the conversation, he dismissed with good-humoured disbelief. There being no past history of any sexual deviation, and no present signs of any mental illness, the psychiatrist concluded that there was nothing for him to do, and that it was up to the police to take legal action if they saw fit.

However, the matter did not rest there. It was said that yet again Mr Graham had been found in a compromising position with a child, and this after being begged and warned by his children and the home help to keep away from little girls in the park at all costs. So strong was public feeling against the old man that the street rose up and demanded his removal. The home help tried to stick by him, but felt that by doing so she came in for the same hostility. The police were pressured and they in turn pressed the psychiatrist, who reluctantly consented to admit the old chap for assessment into a psychiatric ward if he would agree to come in. He did, and left his home for ever.

In the hospital, over a period of several weeks, he showed no features of mental disorder. In that setting there was, of course, no scope for whatever may have been his sexual proclivities. A place was eventually found for him in an old people's home near one of his children, and he was discharged there in the hope that there would be no more trouble, and that he would settle down happily. Although it seemed very likely that the reports of him were true, they were never confirmed, and he was never convicted. While everyone was acting for the best, Mr Graham lost his home, his reputation and his way of life by means which would never have been countenanced in a younger man. He also lost heart. The home was not at all keen on having a sexual offender among its residents, and he was not made welcome, his freedom to go out was curtailed, and he pined. He was transferred to another home, and another, before moves were made to get him back into the hospital again. It was not that he had done anything to warrant readmission, but the homes' staffs shared the attitudes of his neighbourhood, and in such a situation the only place where he could find asylum was— The Asylum. However, before he could be shifted yet again, he died.

Incontinence, one of the least socially acceptable disabilities of old age, is not confined to those who are demented or have urinary tract infection or mechanical faults rendering them unable to hold their water. There are similarities between urinary incontinence in the elderly and bed-wetting children, and although physical causes are far more common in the former, psychological factors should not be forgotten. For instance occasionally incontinence, like bed-wetting, is comprehensible as a way of 'hitting back' by someone who is in too subordinate and dependent a position to do so in a more direct manner. Apathy, arising from depression, malaise, loss of self-respect and lack of stimulation, frequently accompanies and contributes to incontinence.

Apathy most often arises from mental disorder (depression, dementia) or debilitating physical illness, but can be a problem in its own right. Apathetic old people sit about, and are game for nothing. They stare into space, or snooze most of the day. They are early to bed and late to rise. Many seem quite content to be totally unoccupied, provided they get their meals and are kept warm and comfortable. Apathy is a major challenge to institutions for the elderly, where so many people sit round the walls, waiting to be fed and put to bed. While the lack of occupation where staff are short contributes to the apathy, there is no denying that a high proportion of old people who stay in an institution are pretty apathetic anyway, and it is a tough job to arouse and sustain their interest even in the liveliest unit. There is a world of difference between the members of the average Darby and Joan Club and the patients in their local geriatric or psychogeriatric ward, or even the residents of the nearby old people's home. The differences is not just because those in the club are healthier, or because of the demoralising effects of institutionalisation, but also because apathetic old people seem more likely to drift into institutional care. Among them are those who have given up the struggle with ageing and surrendered to a 'living death' which they do not find uncongenial.

Hypochondria has been mentioned several times in previous chapters, as a common symptom of depression and anxiety states. Hypochondriacs, however, may be just that, without any other evidence of psychiatric disorder. They enjoy, as has been said, 'the best of bad health'; their multitudinous symptoms have become part of their personalities, sometimes their raison d'être. For the lonely, the condition is a season ticket to medical consultations and the companionship of a doctor's waiting room and outpatient departments. For the insignificant, their mysterious and incurable malady is a conversation piece, a status symbol and an object of sympathy. For the disgruntled and resentful the affliction is one which may be used to afflict others. (It has been said that in middle-age psychopaths tend to turn into hypochondriacs.) These forms of 'secondary gain' do nto explain the development of the symptoms in the first place, but often account for the tenacity with which the hypochondriac clings to them; indeed, it is often evident that even if it were possible to take the symptoms away, it would be an unkindness to do so. In the elderly, hypochondria usually focuses on constipation; the bowel becomes the centre of their being.

Anorexia nervosa in which young women starve and purge themselves to conform to their somewhat bizarre body image of the shape and weight they would like to be, and stop menstruating, may be represented in later life by old ladies, neither, it seems, depressed nor physically ill, but often hypochondriacal about their insides, who eat alarmingly little and reach body weights as low as 25 kg (4 stone). In one patient this self-destructive tendency related, it seemed, to her husband's suicide many years ago, and there was a clear sexual imagery to her hypochondriasis: 'There's all white stuff coming away from me'. The condition is difficult to check, and readily proves fatal.

Addiction, to alcohol or drugs, is much less common in old age than in early adulthood and middle age—partly because alcoholism and addiction in no way promote longevity. Most elderly alcoholics have somehow survived as such for many years, but some old people take to drink as a consolation for loneliness. Old ladies sometimes tipple cream sherry or tonic wine, or down Guinness 'for the sake of their health', to an extent which is not appreciated until a visit to the home reveals a large number of empty bottles beneath the sink; the cause of the bouts of confusion and staggering is then apparent. Abuse of drugs is more often due to absent-mindedness than addiction but dependency on sleeping tablets (for instances barbiturates) is all too common, and can be a cause of confusion, depression and debility. The elderly should not be the greatest consumers of hypnotics, but they are.

Management

Strictly there is no treatment for personality disorder. 'What can't be cured must be endured', and management is directed towards acceptance of this harsh fact of life. When vain hopes of cure or change are relinquished, the task of adjusting to the inevitable can begin.

Old people need to accept what they are, and those dealing with them must take the rough with the smooth, the sow's ears with silk purses, without hoping to change the one into the other, *Acceptance* mitigates personality disorder, while rejection aggravates it. The transfer of awkward old people from home to hospital, from ward to ward, then from home to home and then, perhaps, back to hospital again, is thoughtless and cruel. Small wonder that after such an experience the unfortunate victim of his own temperament and other's intolerance will settle nowhere except, perhaps, in the haven of a mental hospital. But mental hospitals are not the answer to the problem of the unbiddable aged. Their days may be numbered and their beds are needed for those who are ill, and not for the misfits. Every agency concerned with the elderly should expect to cope with its share of difficult customers, without trying to pass them on to somebody else. Advice may reasonably be sought on whether there is any place for treatment, and on how to cope with the problem, but not on to whom to pass the buck.

To be accepted, warts and all, can be immensely reassuring to a disturbed personality. The personality will not change, but behaviour gradually becomes more appropriate to the situation. There will be periodic disruptions, often occasioned by changes or upsets in the surroundings which will be tested out by a return to the old pattern of protest, but if the response is tolerant and understanding, equilibrium is soon restored.

For the 'patient', *support*, along the lines described in previous chapters, may be appropriate, if he can allow a relationship at all. Drugs however, have a very limited place, and when given are prescribed more often to satisfy the needs of others that something should be seen to be given than for any benefit there is likely to be to him.

Support is also needed by those who deal with the personality disordered—families, friends (if any) and workers within the community and the institutions. This may be given, according to the situation, by the doctor, social worker, ward sister, matron or warden of an old people's home, or those to whom they are responsible. The psychiatrist often has a role here, provided he is not looked upon as the man with the answer (or the bed to which the 'problem' can be removed) Support mainly consists of not merely allowing but actively encouraging the off-loading of all the hostile feelings which are focused on this troublesome old person. 'Blowing off steam' like this discharges frustrated resentment, restores perspective (frequently it will be recognised that some of the anger arises from grievances which really have nothing to do with the old person at all) and eases the burden of care. Frank meetings among family or staff are helpful; the sharing of negative feelings relieves individual guilt, and after a good 'hate' session good humour is regained and more constructive attitudes are strengthened.

Operant conditioning may modify the more disturbing, disruptive or disgusting forms of behaviour disorder by somehow rewarding its avoidance and not its indulgence. For example, a lady who picked her nose vigorously and made revolting noises at mealtimes yet craved company was consistently isolated when she behaved in this manner, but rewarded with a cosy table for two with a favoured nurse when she did not (see also Ch. 7 and 15.)

REFERENCES

Macmillan D, Shaw P 1966 Senile Breakdown in standards of personal and environmental cleanliness. Brit Med J 2: 1032

12

A psychogeriatric service

The principle aim of a psychogeriatric service must be to meet the needs of the old people in its community. Usually the service operates from the psychiatric hospital or unit for the area, but it is concerned not merely or even mostly with those old people already in hospital, but with the development of comprehensive assessment, treatment and care for the elderly mentally ill at large.

It may first be helpful to consider the characteristics of an *unorganised* psychogeriatric service:

This is likely to be bed-orientated. There will be many beds—too many for the staff and space available—occupied by elderly patients, mainly women. A few will be acutely ill, on admission wards taking patients of all ages, or perhaps in a special admission ward for the elderly, taking predominantly confused patients. Some of these will die (usually of pneumonia) within three months. Others may not be ill at all, but will have recovered from whatever symptoms they had at the time of the crisis precipitating their admission. They either lack the drive and will to seek their discharge, or there are obstacles such as the lack of suitable accommodation to go to, or rejection by their families. 'Part Three accommodation' (in old people's homes) may have been sought on their behalf, but very few go there unless there is a swap with someone the home badly wishes to get away. The nurses, however, are quite glad to have these patients on their wards, for they are very little trouble.

Many more of the hospital's elderly patients will be severely demented, often with associated behaviour disturbance—wandering, incontinence, destructiveness and aggression. They may be collected together on wards for the demented, or scattered among the chronic wards, among the hospital's many elderly schizophrenics, as beds have fallen vacant. And finally, there will be a sizeable number of infirm patients, physically ill and bedridden, with bedsores, on sick wards where the nursing is especially heavy.

Patients accepted for admission are, particularly if confused, placed at the end of a lengthy waiting list. Little will be known about them, or about which of them are in greatest need. Some, when sent for after a delay of weeks or months, will have died. Any relief, on the hospital's part, is unjustified, for the service has failed: deaths on the waiting list suggest either that there was an important factor of physical illness which should have been diagnosed so that proper treatment could have been arranged elsewhere, or that the patient died of neglect. By the time the surviving patients are admitted after this long wait it is not expected by their families, GPs, the community or indeed the hospital itself that they will ever be discharged home.

None of the senior psychiatrists will have a primary commitment to the elderly; indeed, they will give far less of their time to them than to younger patients, and may even resent the little time they do give. Visits to patients' homes, for assessment after they have been referred, will be few and perfunctory. A succession of junior doctors, with scant supervision, will look after the old people who are admitted. Some of these doctors will be energetic and imaginative, others bored and idle, but they will work independently, without sharing their experience. There will be no on-going policy, and liaison with the local geriatricians and social services will be poor. These and other agents, including the general practitioners and families, will be regarded with dark suspicion as all too ready to exploit and over-burden the hospital, giving nothing in return.

There will be good nurses on the psychogeriatric wards, but they will feel that they are not appreciated, are working on their own, and that if there are any complaints, they will get the blame. Otherwise the allocation of the hospital's resources to the elderly will be meagre. An overworked part-time social worker will do her best with an impossible load. Psychogeriatric patients will rarely visit the occupational therapy department, and occupational therapists will rarely visit those wards. There may or may not be some sporadic, haphazard physiotherapy (usually the hospital will not have been able to attract the services of a physiotherapist) and voluntary visiting. (Volunteers will be given a cool reception, as potentially troublesome do-gooders who will create more work than they will ever.)

The wards will be the least attractive in the hospital. Most patients will rarely leave them. They will be totally unoccupied. They will lack personal lockers in which to keep their belongings. Their glasses, false teeth and hearing aids will have been mislaid or stored away. Aids to walking will not be available, and patients will, indeed, be discouraged from walking. The ward will be up one or two flights of stairs, with no lift. Washing facilities will be meagre, and the lavatories cold, damp and dirty. Most patients will be incontinent. They will go to bed early (from 5 p.m. onwards) and be kept in bed a good 12 hours, well sedated so that the night nurse will not have too hectic a time; there will not always be a night nurse. Visiting hours will be severely restricted, and once the visitors have left, the ward door will be locked firmly behind them.

Weighed down by its oppressive psychogeriatric load, the hospital will feel angry and impotent. It may even be the subject of one of the periodic 'scandals' which can befall any such institutions when relatives or disenchanted staff bring negligence or actual ill treatment to light. After investigation a few heads may roll and there may even be a drastic reorganisation, but just as often attitudes are even more entrenched and bitter than before.

To change this unhappy state of affairs (which I have by. no means exaggerated or caricatured) and establish an *effective* psychogeriatric service the following need to be established:

1. A psychogeriatric team
2. Assessment before admission
3. Active liaison

THE PSYCHOGERIATRIC TEAM

There is much to be said for creating within the psychiatric hospital or department a team (or 'firm') entirely concerned with the psychiatry of old age. In the first place this improves the organisation of resources within the hospital, and gives those working with the elderly a sense of identity. The firm becomes a focus for the efforts of those who want to improve the lot of the older patients, and a powerful voice within the hospital community. Ultimately as all work together the waiting list and death rate diminish, while the discharge rate increases. Tables 3 and 4 demonstrate the effects of establishing a psychogeriatric firm at Claybury Hospital in 1966. Arie (1971) published figures showing the same trends even more strikingly after the creation of a similar firm at the nearby Goodmayes Hospital (both are on the fringe of London, in Essex) in 1969. Conditions for the elderly in the hospital improve, experience and knowledge increase, and more staff are attracted.

The team is led by a consultant psychiatrist with a major (though not necessarily exclusive) committment to psychogeriatrics. In 1966 there were only one or two consultants in such posts in Great Britain. In 1973 there were almost 30, and a special Group for the Psychiatry of Old Age was set up within the Royal College of

Table 3   Claybury psychogeriatric firm

		Admissions, discharges and deaths, 1964–68			
Year	1964	1965	1966	1967	1968
Admissions	360	378	428	441	412
	♀243 ♂117	♀266 ♂112	♀295 ♂133	♀308 ♂133	♀266 ♂146
Discharges (as percentage of admissions)	231	203	295	331	325
	64%	54%	69%	76%	79%
Deaths (percentage of admissions)	168	202	208	168	129
	47%	53%	49%	38%	31%
Excess of deaths and discharges over admissions	39	27	75	63	42

Note. Marked increase in admissions after establishment of the firm, but greatly increased proportion of discharges to admissions in 1967 and 1968, and an excess of departures over admissions every year, before and after the firm's creation, but attributable more to discharges than deaths in 1967 and 1968. Trends were, however, maintained without increasing in 1968; indeed, there was slight drop in the discharge rate and increase in the death rate. In that year the service had reached the limit of its resources. These were therefore increased by the creation of a second psychogeriatric firm in 1969.

Table 4   Some comparisons between admissions and their outcome (in the following year) in 1964 and 1967 (i.e. shortly before and shortly after the establishment of a psychogeriatric firm at Claybury)

	1964	*1967*
Total admissions	358	413
Discharged home or to old people's home	156 (44%)	248 (60%)
Discharged to general hospital	29	32
Died	83	79
Remained in hospital over 1 year	88	51
Disposal other than above	2	3
Readmitted	48(30% of b)	97 (40% of b)
Assessment before admission: domiciliary visit	28	130
outpatient	61 (40%)	64 (63%)
social worker	55	66

Note. There were almost twice as many readmissions in 1967 as in 1964 but even so, there were nearly 50 more patients discharged in 1967 who did not return.

The increased proportion of assessments before admission in 1967 is almost entirely made up of domiciliary visits, of which there were more than four times as many as in 1964.

Psychiatrists. Five years later, when the Group applied to the College for full recognition as a section, there were one hundred consultant members with a special concern for the elderly, approximately ten per cent of the country's consultants in adult psychiatry (Wattis et al, 1981).

Doubts that it would be possible to attract doctors of the necessary calibre have generally been dispelled. Psychogeriatrics is, after all, a fascinating speciality, demanding the full range of psychiatric skills and a good knowledge of general and social medicine. The 'psychogeriatrician' soon has special skills to impart, which doctors in training wish to acquire in order to have a full grounding in psychiatry and thus the medical team builds up.

The other members of the team are the nurses, social workers, psychologists, occupational therapists and physiotherapists.

It is important that the team deal with *all* referrals of patients over 65, and not just the confused, physically disabled and obviously aged. Thus the firm does not feel burdened by an almost entirely chronic and irrecoverable clientele, but also treats many patients, especially those with functional illness, such as depression, who can be discharged cured or greatly improved. Thus there is a steady turnover in a good half of the admission ward beds, and often it seems that because of this some of the less likely prospects for discharge are able to go home too. The atmosphere and attitudes on a ward where patients are always coming and going are very different from those on a ward with an almost static population. It is sometimes argued that people should not be shunted into a psychogeriatric service, away from the company of younger folk, because they happen to be over 65. While I have some sympathy with this view, it is my experience that such patients are only allowed to have one or two episodes of illness in a general psychiatric ward before being passed to the psychogeriatrician anyway—at the age of 68 or 69 instead of 65—so they might as well have come into the hands of those who are going to go on dealing with them for the rest of their lives in the first place. The psychogeriatric firm is glad to have these patients and will treat them no less effectively than a general psychiatric firm; indeed, being specialists in the problems of the over 65s (who all have in common that they are of retiring age and, like it or not, facing a period of decline) they may even do a little better.

Tables 5–8 illustrate the work of the psychogeriatric service based upon the London Hospital (St Clement's) during the year 1979/80. Table 6, which lists the diagnoses of those referred, shows how, once such a firm is established, organic illness accounts for less than half the referrals.

Table 5 Sources of referrals to the London Hospital Psychogeriatric Service during 12 months from 1st April 1979–31st March 1980 (percentages in parenthesis)

General practitioner	185	(44)
General physician	54	(13)
Geriatrician	44	(11)
Social worker or health visitor	35	(8)
Psychiatrist	29	(7)
Community nurse	25	(6)
Matron of residential home	16	(4)
Patient's relative	12	(3)
Police	6	(>1)
Surgeon	5	(>1)
Warden (of sheltered housing)	3	(<1)
Self referral	3	(<1)
Voluntary worker	2	(>0)
Total	419	(100)

Table 6 Diagnoses of patients referred to the London Hospital Psychogeriatric Service during 12 months from 1st April 1979 to 31st March 1980 (percentages in parenthesis)

Confusional state	58		(14)	
Dementia	103	161	(25)	(39)
Depressive illness	135		(32)	
Mania and hypomania	6		(>1)	
Paranoid state (paraphrenia)	37		(9)	
Schizophrenia	16		(4)	
Anxiety state	5		(>1)	
Obsessional neurosis	1		(>0)	
Personality and behaviour disorder	42		(10)	
Marital problem	4		(1)	
Physical disorder only	6		(>1)	
(Significant physical disorder complicating psychiatric disorder above)		51		(12)
No psychiatric disability	6		(>1)	
Total	419		(99)	

The Department of Health and Social Security has recommended that there should be provided one bed for 'functional' illness for every 2000 of the population over 65, and five to six beds for those with severe dementia.

In most general hospital psychiatric units at present there are nowhere near this number of beds for the elderly, while in the mental hospitals there may be more. It is hoped that the combination of modern treatment and community care will reduce the number of psychiatric patients of all ages, including the elderly, so

Table 7   Initial assessment of patients referred to the London Hospital Psychogeriatric Service during 12 months from 1st April 1979–31st March 1980 (percentages in parenthesis)

Visited at home (house call)	305	(73)
Visited in general or geriatric hospital	84	(20)
Outpatient consultation	28	(7)
Telephone consultation	2	(>0)
Total	419	(100)

Table 8   Action taken after initial assessment of patients referred to the London Hospital Psychogeriatric Service during 12 months from 1st April 1979–31st March 1980 (percentages in parenthesis)

Admitted to psychogeriatric ward	109	(26)
functional	78	(19)
dementia		
holiday	5	(>1)
continuing care	3	(<1)
joint unit in general hospital	21	(5)
other psychiatric ward hospital	2	(>0)
Admitted to psychogeriatric day hospital	88	(21)
lower dependency (mainly functional)	62	(15)
higher dependency (mainly demented)	26	(6)
Referred to geriatrician	12	(3)
Referred to other specialist	6	(>1)
Residential home recommended	17	(4)
Referred to local authority day centre	9	(2)
Personal social services increased	7	(<2)
Medication prescribed/modified only	37	(9)
Outpatient follow up	15	(<4)
Review (usually by community psychogeriatric nurse)	39	(9)
Advice/reassurance given only	47	(11)
No action thought necessary	23	(>5)
Refused help offered	6	(>1)
Died before action taken	4	(1)
Total	419	(99)

that the bed allocation recommended will suffice. It has been anticipated that the mental hospitals will eventually be closed, that acutely ill patients will be treated in the psychiatric and psychogeriatric units of the large district general hospitals, and demented patients will be cared for in the smaller and less comprehensive community hospitals, as near as possible to their homes.

Meanwhile, in the mental hospital which may well have as many as 20 wards with predominantly or entirely elderly patients, it is a good idea to separate the 'graduates', i.e. those who came into the hospital, usually with schizophrenia, many years ago and have grown old without ever having left. These are not, strictly, psychogeriatric patients and should be looked after by the other firms. The remainder, i.e. those who have been admitted with psychiatric disorder developing or recurring after the age of 65 (and forming 50 to 60 per cent of all the old people in the hospital) should be in wards at ground level or with lifts, as near as possible to a central administrative office, where the receptionist, secretaries, nursing officers, senior social worker and occupational therapist and the consultant are stationed. There, should be one or two admission wards (preferably one for 'organic' the other for 'functional' patients, as their needs are different—Table 8) follow-on (rehabilitation), continuing care and sick wards. These wards should be mixed, with male and female patients and a mixed staff. It is natural for men and women to live together, and socially they stimulate each other, whereas segregation of the sexes hastens the deadening process of institutionalisation. There should be regular meetings of all who work on the firm to discuss their work, new developments and difficulties, and to promote education.

A day hospital, either within the psychiatric hospital or preferably placed nearer to the patients' homes in a general hospital, is a very desirable, if not an essential facility. It offers a real alternative to admission, promotes discharges and offers continuing support to many patients who would otherwise relapse and have to be readmitted again and again (see Ch.16).

ASSESSMENT BEFORE ADMISSION

It should be the aim of the psychogeriatric service to assess every unknown old person referred for admission before he or she is accepted. Assessment after admission is of far less importance—the decision *whether* to admit at all is much more vital than *where*.

If the hospital staff remain embattled within the institutional walls, trying to fend off elderly patients who are likely to remain and require a lot of nursing, they really deserve to be stuck with those who slip beneath their guard.

Much the best assessment, in my opinion, is by a domiciliary visit, made usually by the consultant psychiatrist, accompanied by one or two members of the team. He is thus enabled to see the patient at home, and meet the family, neighbours, social worker and (with luck) the general practitioner concerned. It is instructive to see the house itself, and the neighbourhood. Thus it is possible to make the correct social diagnosis, which is often more important then the ostensible medical diagnosis on the strength of which the patient was referred, and make appropriate recommendations. General practitioners welcome such visits without feeling that their word is being doubted or their territory invaded once they appreciate that the aim is to use the hospital beds for those who are found to need them most, and give aid and advice for those who do not need admission.

Table 8 shows how patients referred to the London Hospital psychogeriatric service are assessed. Over 70 per cent receive a domiciliary visit. Those in other hospitals are assessed in those hospitals, and only ten per cent of all those referred are initially seen in St Clement's Hospital as outpatients. This is possible because the catchment area is compact, and because the whole working of the firm is geared to domiciliary appraisal.

Only 26 per cent were in fact admitted to the psychiatric hospital, but satisfactory alternative management was arranged for most of the rest. Those who were accepted for admission came in soon enough—within 24 hours as a rule and a week at the most. Consequently very few indeed died while still waiting for appropriate action to be taken.

There is no denying that the committment to a policy of domiciliary assessment is exacting as well as rewarding, but in my opinion it is a sine qua non for an effective psychogeriatric service, and consequently nobody should take up psychogeriatrics who is not prepared to spend a great deal of time out of hospital and in patients' homes. Those admitted are not usually accepted for long-term care (though of course, a few stay). At the time of the home visit it is stated that admission is for treatment, with a view to return home in an improved condition.

Outpatient consultations in psychogeriatric clinics held in general hospitals are another useful means of assessment before admission. The facilities for physical investigations to some extent offset the disadvantage of not seeing the patient at home. However, if outpatient assessment is to be of much value emergency appointments must always be available.

Assessment in a *day hospital* is a third and useful means, the patient's behaviour and response to the environment being observed over the course of one or more days rather than the mere half to one hour available for domiciliary and outpatient assessment.

ACTIVE LIAISON

Liaison means getting to know the other workers in the field and the jobs they have to do, so that all can work effectively together. Perhaps the hardest task in liaison is to appreciate that the others have problems to contend with quite as big as our own. It is much easier to blame than to make the effort to understand the others' difficulties.

The Department of Health in Great Britain (1970) set great store by *psychogeriatric assessment units,* recommending that about one bed for every 2000 old people should be provided for this purpose. Perhaps the greatest advantage of these units is that those key workers in the field who provide institutional services, the geriatrician, the psychiatrist and, it is to be hoped, the officer responsible for the local authority's residential homes for the elderly, can meet regularly on common ground—especially if, as in the unit which used to operate off St Francis Hospital in Nottingham, all have the right to admit.

It is now recognised that 'misplacement' of psychiatric patients in geriatric wards and vice versa is not as widespread as was feared after a report published some years ago (Kidd, 1962) which failed to allow for the high proportion of geriatric patients discharged or dead three weeks after their admission, when the survey was made. Nor, despite the great differences between geriatric and psychogeriatric wards in their emphasis on physical treatment and rehabilitation, are the effects of any misplacement on the patient's progress and chances of survival very marked (Mezey, Hodkinson & Evans, 1968). Any misplacement is particularly unlikely to occur in a service which makes frequent home assessments. So for this purpose the assessment unit is superfluous.

The units are sited in the district general hospitals as part of the geriatric department. While the geriatrician and psychiatrist both have beds, the former is likely to be officially in charge of the running of the ward. As many as possible of the nurses should have a psychiatric as well as a general nursing qualification. A social worker, occupational therapist and physiotherapist form the rest of the team, while at a weekly ward round attended by both the consultants, representatives of the community workers—the Social Services Department, district nurse, health visitors and perhaps a GP or two—should also be present, to look at the patients in the unit together, and in collaboration work out the best means of helping them.

The most suitable patients for the assessment unit are those:

1. Suffering from acute confusional state (delirium)—the physical cause for which is obviously best treated in a general hospital.

2. Suspected to be suffering dementia, and requiring investigation to eliminate alternatives.

3. Suffering from serious psychiatric and physical disorder at the same time, e.g. depression and heart failure, mania and pneumonia.

4. Showing symptoms the cause of which is not clear before admission, e.g. immobility and falls, and failure to thrive (which is all that the term senility means) which can be due to physical or psychiatric disease, or both.

There are obvious advantages to physically ill psychiatric patients in having access to the facilities of a general hospital—laboratory investigations, X-rays, occupational therapy and physiotherapy in particular. Geriatric patients with psychological problems are likewise bound to benefit from the more reflective, enquiring, tolerant and patient-orientated approach of the psychiatric staff.

It has been suggested that in association with the assessment unit there should be an office to which all problems affecting old people who are unable to cope at home might be referred. This office would then be the hub of the geriatric, psychogeriatric and social services for the elderly. The separation of social from health services in Britain has made the full realisation of this suggestion unlikely, but the London Hospital, for example, has an office, adjacent to the psychogeriatric assessment unit, to which all requests for the admission of elderly patients from the borough of Tower Hamlets may be referred. It has been found that this saves the general practitioner the problem of deciding whether to refer his patient to the geriatrician or psychiatrist, and saves the duplication of effort where previously a patient was referred to each in turn, with no mention of the fact that the other had already been consulted.

Patients should not remain in the assessment unit for longer than a month, for otherwise there will not be sufficient turnover for the unit to serve its purpose. Most will be discharged home, some will die, and others will be moved to other accommodation, in a geriatric or psychiatric ward or an old people's home. Clearly, if the unit is to work effectively, there must be enough alternative accommodation for those patients deemed to have need of it at the end of their month. Details of particular units are given by Arie & Dunn (1973), and Pitt & Silver (1980), while Godber (1978) has written a valuable review of the subject.

Where there is no assessment unit, an arrangement whereby the psychiatrist and geriatrician visit patients in each other's wards is a very satisfactory alternative. Again, this not only makes the expertise of each available to a wider range of patients but promotes liaison between two specialists who must work closely together to ensure that the best use is made of available resources.

Attendance by community workers at rounds is just as desirable in the psychogeriatric wards of the mental hospital as at the assessment unit. Then not only can all the information known about the patients under discussion be shared with the hospital staff, but the workers within and without the hospital are enabled to know and respect each other.

A particularly inspiring model for liaison has been the Department of Health Care of the Elderly at Nottingham University, which combines geriatrics and psychiatry under a professor (Tom Aire) who happens to be a psychiatrist, with senior lecturers (associate professors) and consultants in both specialties working in separate wards within the same building with a great deal of cross consultation, conferring as a department and providing an integrated course for medical students.

Arie's aim is to provide a comprehensive service so that once referred the patient's needs will be met by and generally within the department by the range of experts and specialists available, without any referral back to look elsewhere for help.

Active liaison means taking every opportunity to meet and talk with the many other workers in the field of psychogeriatrics—at staff meetings, on home visits, in committees, over the 'phone, and socially. It means dropping prejudices, removing blinkers and not passing the buck. It involves giving help and claiming it, talking and listening, and the flexible use of persuasion, assertion, enlightenment and at times even anger, provided that afterwards communication survives.

REFERENCES

Arie T 1971 Morale and planning of psychogeriatric services. Brit Med J 3: 166
Arie T, Dunn T 1973 A 'do it yourself' psychiatric/geriatric joint patient unit. Lancet 2: 1313
Department of Health and Social Security 1970 N H S psychogeriatric assessment units. HM(70)11
Department of Health and Social Security 1972 Services for mental illness related to old age. HM(72)71
Godber C 1978 Conflict and collaboration between geriatric medicine and psychiatry. In: Isaacs B (ed.) Recent advances in geriatric medicine. Churchill Livingstone, Edinburgh
Kidd 1962 Misplacement of the elderly in hospital. Brit Med J 2: 1491
Mezey A, Hodkinson H M, Evans G 1968 The elderly in the wrong unit. Brit Med J 2: 967
Pitt B, Silver C P 1980 The combined approach to geriatrics and psychiatry: evaluation of a joint unit in a teaching hospital district. Age and Ageing?
Wattis J, Wattis L, Arie T 1981 Psychogeriatrics: a national survey of a new branch of psychiatry. Brit Med J 1: 1529

13

Principles of treatment

Prevention is (to coin a phrase) better than cure. However, the place for *primary* prevention (i.e. measures to stop old people from becoming mentally ill) in psychogeriatrics is not at all clear. The losses associated with ageing (and described in Ch. 2) must contribute to the high incidence of *depression*, though, and some measures to render them less overwhelming will therefore be briefly considered.

Loss of *status* may be to some extent offset by *education* to promote a more humane and favourable attitude towards the aged and ageing, based at the very least upon enlightened self-interest, the elderly not being regarded so much as 'them', but as 'us' a few years hence. Education within the 'caring' professions is especially vital to enable future doctors, nurses and social workers to understand how much old people need their services, and how rewarding the work with them can be.

The preparations for retirement organised by some of the larger firms, local authorities and voluntary bodies should be of value in helping some people to develop interests which will sustain them when they would otherwise have nothing to do, and to make sensible plans for when income is reduced and health fails, but probably those who most need such instruction are least likely to avail themselves of it; instead they will 'deny' the fact of retirement until it has overtaken them.

It would be better to ensure that everyone who so wishes can *work* past retiring age, at least some of the time. If this were extensively applied the implications for the employment of younger workers would have to be thrashed out in Parliament; a climate of unemployment is hardly conducive to such a rearrangement of work. On the other hand, there are some who might wish to retire earlier, say at 60, or even 55, so some flexibility might be brought to the arrangement. A few large firms have facilities for their old employees to do perhaps a day's work a week past retirement age, and some local authorities have special workshops for the elderly.

In Canada an employee has already successfully challenged his retirement on the grounds that it is ageist and discriminatory.

The ability of some old people to *help others* should be exploited to the full, e.g. as home helps and paid 'good neighbours' to the more frail elderly and young parents. This role for the healthy 'senior citizen' is highly appropriate and badly needs promotion.

Loss of *income* is inevitable, but the effects of inflation should be met by much more flexible adjustments of pensions in proportion to rises in the cost of living, though the cost is daunting for countries, like Britain, with a struggling economy. More money needs to be spent on services for the elderly. In Britain this is currently taking the form of reallocation of some money spent on the so called 'acute' health services for the elderly and mentally ill, though this is mainly a redistribution of hospital beds. Again, the Medicare programme in the United States is for those who are already ill.

Loss of *physical health* can be mitigated by a positive health programme. Dietary education helps the best use of slender means, and may prevent malnutrition and obesity. Dining clubs and Meals on Wheels also help to maintain nutrition. Glasses, hearing aids and dentures need to be provided early, for it is hard to teach an older dog new tricks. Cigarette smoking, which contributes to lung cancer, bronchitis and heart disease needs to be actively discouraged. Geriatric or pre-geriatric welfare clinics, providing health checks for those approaching old age, may detect disorders such as diabetes and hypertension early and treatment may then be more effective than later. The maintenance of an 'at risk' register of those over 70, already infirm, or newly bereaved or rehoused, who would be regularly visited by, say, a health visitor attached to a general practice, is likely to be a valuable means of identifying illness before it has gone too far. Safety measures should be taken in the home to reduce the risk of accidents, e.g. rails where stairs are steep, non-slip rugs and proper lighting.

The loss of *company* can be met, to some extent, by the provision of other company. Home visiting may be very acceptable to some lonely old people, provided that the same person calls regularly and does not take a patronising attitude; there is great scope for volunteers here. (Note to prospective visitors: always accept the cup of tea offered—you will hurt your host's feelings if you do not, and however anxious you may be about how hygenically it was prepared it probably will not kill you!) Day clubs and day centres provide social activity for the more extraverted. The bereaved are in particular need of comfort and support.

The harmful effects of the loss of *independence* because of infirmity can at least be reduced by a regard for the old person's basic psychological needs for respect, security and self-determination (see pp. 21–22).

The problems of unsuitable *accomodation* require an imaginative and flexible housing policy, in which warden-supervised flatlets, 'three-generation' homes (giving the grandparent a self-contained flat adjacent to her children) and old people's homes all have a place. Warden-supervision can be arranged in housing estates for old people who do not choose to live with other old people. The disadvantages of disrupting the extended family need to be examined critically—if daughter moves out to Harlow, what will become of Nan in Bethnal Green? (Or, sometimes, as I have found, what will happen to the daughter in Harlow, who no longer has her mother to turn to?) At the same time, it is often unwise to house old people with their children—a little home of their own nearby may be preferable. Moves away from a familiar neighbourhood are undesirable unless there is a great need to be near children who are at a distance. Preparation for, and support through, rehousing are important, for at first the move may be seen as more of a blow than a boon.

For those who must remain in their old homes, improvements, safety measures and, for the disabled, aids to daily living (such as a handle on the lavatory wall for those who find it difficult to get themselves up) should be more readily installed than is often the case now.

The Church can help a lot with the spiritual problems associated with *dying*, but doctors, nurses, social workers and families need to be much franker about and less afraid of the subject of death. The final leave-taking should be avoided less often, and the feelings of the bereaved faced. The development of the 'hospice' movement in Britain, associated particularly with the names of Dame Cecily Saunders and Drs Colin Murray Parkes and Lammerton, has done much to improve the care and understanding of the dying.

All these measures improve the quality of life in old age, and might reduce the frequency of depressive disorders. But, as Dr Felix Post has remarked (Post, 1965), isolating and alienating personality traits operating throughout a lifetime, constitutional factors determining psychosis and organic deterioration causing confusion and dementia are hardly likely to be modified greatly by these means. For these primary prevention gives place to *secondary* prevention—reducing the duration of established disorder by effective identification and treatment—and *tertiary* prevention—using *re-*

habilitation to enable patients to make the best use of their residual abilities.

The first step in effective treatment is *early diagnosis*. So often, as has been stated earlier, help is demanded at a time of crisis after prolonged illness, when considerable damage has already been done to the patient's self-confidence and her relations with her family, neighbours and the supportive services. It may then be that specific treatment of the illness, though successful, is followed by rejection or relapse.

In the past too many doctor's education in the psychiatry of old age stopped short at senile dementia. There is a great need for proper instruction and practical experience in this field, not only for medical but also for nursing and social work students. It is not possible to diagnose that of which one is unaware.

There is little point, either, in making a diagnosis if it will not lead to some useful action on the patients' behalf. There is a greater incentive to early diagnosis in areas where there is an efficient psychogeriatric service (see previous chapter). Outpatient or, better still, domiciliary consultations (as so often social circumstances are of prime importance) improve the accuracy of diagnosis and quality of treatment. If the mental hospital is seen as the source of the psychogeriatric service, and not just as a repository for those dements whom the geriatrician and the old people's homes will not take, the attitude of 'do not go in till the last possible moment, because when you do go in you go for good' will change, and admission for treatment and return home be considered more favourably.

The general practitioner needs to be in regular, frequent contact with those of his elderly patients who are 'at risk' (see p. 143), and those who do not 'bother' him at the surgery need to be visited at home. An extra financial allowance for elderly patients on the doctor's list may be an inducement, but better still is the attachment of a nurse or health visitor to the practice for the purpose.

After early diagnosis, the second principle of treatment is to enable the elderly patient to *stay in her own home* as much and for as long as possible, provided that neither she nor those caring for her suffer unduly. Not only do the elderly on the whole fare far better if not taken away from home, but the shortage of staff to provide custodial care means that this must be reserved for those who really need it— the severely disabled and those who lack the family and community resources to live outside institutions.

This principle does not mean, of course, that admission is to be avoided at all costs: often the use of a hospital for treatment early in the course of an illness, or a Home to provide a holiday for those caring for a demented old person by taking her in for a week or two, means that the need for long-term custodial care can be eliminated altogether.

The best use, indeed, of hospitals and homes is as a complement to the community services, to provide active treatment, rehabilitation to independence, intermittent and holiday admissions and day care, as well as a 'last refuge' for those who have no other.

The third principle of psychogeriatric treatment is *not to undertreat functionally ill patients, nor overtreat the organically ill*. Considerations of age must not interfere with the proper treatment of severe depression, mania and paraphrenia in the elderly. Doses of antidepressives and tranquillisers should generally be the same as for younger patients suffering similar disorders. It is no kindness to withhold electroplexy from a deeply depressed old person, whose misery needs relief as much as does the pain of terminal cancer, and whose life may otherwise be lost unnecessarily through dehydration, starvation or pneumonia. The possible benefits of psychosurgery for the chronically agitated similarly demand consideration. Although psychoanalysts are reluctant to use their skills and scant resources on those who have reached the age of 40, let alone 65, there is an important place for psychotherapy and case work of some sophistication with elderly neurotics and with the families of patients of all kinds.

On the other hand, drugs should be used sparingly for the confused, with a very clear idea of the purpose for which they are being given. No tranquilliser reduces confusion, and many make it worse. Reduction of agitation and aggression is worthwhile, provided that the price, namely that of inducing drowsiness and enfeeblement, is not too high. Drugs are a poor substitute for exercise and occupation. Knocking out a confused old person for the sake of a household, home or hospital ward is only justifiable if it can be shown that otherwise someone else will suffer worse: even so, it is preferable to effect the patient's transfer to a setting where she can be better tolerated. If a 'placebo' effect on the family, care assistants or nurses is required, then as far as possible nothing stronger than a placebo should be inflicted on the patient; but it is far better, if practicable, to talk the situation out with those who are most bothered about it.

In both groups proper care must be given to nutrition. When wondering whether to tube-feed, one probably should. Sleep disturbances need attention, but recourse to sleeping tablets should not be made lightly. Oversedation causes drowsiness by day (and subsequent wakeful nights), falls, undernourishment, incontinence and bedsores. There is also the danger, to functional patients at home, of drug-dependency (see p. 158).

The *therapeutic community* concept, in which full recognition is given to the therapeutic potential of everyone who comes into contact with the patient, including the other patients, is applicable to psychogeriatrics as to other branches of psychiatry (Pitt, 1972). In practical terms this requires a readiness on the part of the leader of the team to share the treatment with, and be open to communication from, others. Meetings with patients (see Ch. 15) and staff play a very important part in the therapeutic community. At staff meetings (which normally follow ward meetings) new patients are introduced (either in person or by the presentation of a full case history), information about others pooled, treatment, rehabilitation and discharge arrangements discussed, and feelings ventilated pretty freely. All available staff, not just the senior nurses, should attend, and community workers should be made very welcome.

In the next four chapters the subjects of drug and physical treatments, psychotherapy, day and social therapies and rehabilitation will be discussed separately.

REFERENCES

Pitt B 1972 A new deal for old patients. In: Schoenberg E (ed.) A hospital looks at itself. Cassirer, London.
Post F 1965 The clinical psychiatry of late life. Pergamon, London.

14

Drug and physical treatments

DRUGS

The tranquillisers

The term 'tranquilliser' was coined in the early 1950s to describe the action of chlorpromazine (Largactil, then introduced by the French), which was found (at least, in moderate doses) to reduce disturbed behaviour without, like the drugs previously used in psychiatry (barbiturates, bromides, paraldehyde), putting the patient to sleep. However in higher doses, especially in the early stages of treatment, Largactil and drugs like it (the *phenothiazine* tranquillisers) often cause drowsiness. The name 'tranquilliser' is also given to quite a different group of drugs which relieve anxiety without producing troublesome sedation; these are the *benzodiazepines*. The two groups are commonly distinguished by calling the latter *minor*, and the phenothiazines *major* tranquillisers.

Tranquillisers differ from, say, the barbiturates by being relatively safe both as regards dependency and their use for suicide attempts.

These drugs probably do not cure illnesses, but suppress symptoms. The major tranquillisers allay the agitation and disturbance which accompany serious mental illness in the elderly, such as mania, severe depression, paranoia and delirium. Mold tranquillisers relieve anxiety associated with the neuroses, milder depressive illness and stressful situations.

As milder psychiatric disorder is far more common than serious mental illness, the minor tranquillisers are far more often prescribed. Although psychiatrists tend to regard the value of drugs in the treatment of anxiety as less than such measures as support, psychotherapy and manipulation of the environment, general practitioners appear to act as if for them tranquillisers are the treatment of choice. Presumably it takes less time to write a prescription for a patient than to hear him out, and while most doctors recognise the value of taking the trouble to understand the problem, the conditions of general practice favour prescribing, especially when the drug is safe.

Major tranquillisers

The two groups in common use are the phenothiazines and the *butyrophenones*. Chlorpromazine, promazine, thioridazine, trifluoperazine, fluphenazine and flupenthixol belong to the first group and haloperidol to the second.

Chlorpromazine (Largactil), the original tranquilliser, is used in doses of 25–150 mg three or four times a day by mouth, or 25–150 mg at a time by injection.

Promazine (Spine) given in the same dosage has about one-third of the effect of chlorpromazine (following the removal of chlorine from the molecule) and is consequently favoured by many (though not by me) for the elderly.

Thioridazine (Melleril) given in the same dosage as chlorpromazine, has about two-thirds the effect.

Trifluoperazine (Stelazine) is a piperazine derivative of the phenothiazines, and has a very powerful action. 1–2 mg three times a day are given for the treatment of neurotic anxiety, and 10–30 mg a day (as tablets or the spansules, which have a 24-hour action) for paranoid states.

Fluphenazine, another piperazine, is given as 2–20 mg/day by mouth, or as the injections fluphenazine enanthate (Moditen) and fluphenazine decanoate (Modecate), 6–25 mg every two to six weeks.

Flupenthixol is an interesting drug which, when given orally as Fluanxol, 0·5–1 mg twice a day, has an antidepressant effect, while as the depôt injection flupenthixol decanoate (Depixol) 10–40 mg every 1–8 weeks, it serves as a major tranquilliser of particular value (like fluphenazine) for psychotic patients unlikely to comply with oral medication (like paraphrenics).

Haloperidol (Serenace) is given in a dosage of 0·5 mg three times a day for neurotic anxiety, 1–3 mg three or four times a day by mouth for seriously disturbed patients, or 5–10 mg by injection (followed by 10 mg of procyclidine (Kemadrin) to prevent muscular spasms).

There are many more major tranquillisers, including pericyazine (Neulactil), perphenazine (Fentazin), thiopropazate (Dartalan), fluspirilene (Redeptin) and clopenthixol (Clopixol), two more long-acting preparations given by injection, but the above are more than enough to meet the needs of psychogeriatric patients.

These tranquillisers are most effective in all the serious functional psychiatric disorders which befall the elderly with the exception of severe depression, and even this they ease by reducing agitation and paranoia. They are also valuable in calming the delirious, while the treatment of the underlying disorder has yet to take effect.

In emergency situations, when disturbance is acute, e.g. mania and delirium, chlorpromazine or haloperidol by injection are the drugs of choice. Chlorpromazine is more likely to cause drowsiness, and sometimes a considerable drop in blood pressure. Haloperidol is free from side-effects except Parkinsonism and muscle spasms, which are usually quite easily controlled by orphenadrine (Disipal) (50–100 mg three times a day).

Trifluoperazine is especially useful in paranoid states. The drug is well tolerated by paraphrenic patients, but less well tolerated by those whose paranoia arises from confusion. Fluphenazine or Depixol injections are especially useful for paraphrenic patients who will not take oral drugs reliably, though side effects are sometimes troublesome (see below).

Small doses of trifluoperazine and haloperidol are sometimes used as alternatives to the minor tranquillisers in the treatment of anxiety and the neuroses, but otherwise the effectiveness of the major tranquillisers in the treatment of such anxiety is small.

The commoner side-effects of the major tranquillisers are:

1. Drowsiness and confusion (chlorpromazine especially).

2. 'Extrapyramidal' effects, mimicking Parkinsonism—muscular stiffness, tremor and spasms, a mask-like expression, inability to keep still (akathesia, often very hard to distinguish from agitation), sweating and drooling. These are particularly effects of the piperazines and haloperidol. *Tardive dyskinesia*, in which various groups of body muscles but especially those of the lips and mouth are almost always on the move when the patient is awake is unfortunately a not uncommon late reaction to the prescription of phenothiazines, especially in the elderly. It more often follows the use of piperazine derivatives and butyrophenones, i.e. trifluoperazine (Stelazine), the depôt injections and haloperidol and is probably least seen after treatment with thioridazine (Melleril). The condition is at best an unsightly nuisance, often interferes with speech and may cause difficulty in swallowing. As there is no reliably effective treatment-stopping the drug does not stop the dyskinesia —prevention is much better than cure, i.e. these drugs should only be given when, and for as long as, they are absolutely needed.

3. Lowering of blood pressure, e.g. 'Largactil shock'. This is treated by putting the patient to bed and raising the foot of the bed to make sure that the blood has no difficulty in reaching the head.

Occasionally this effect is produced by a small dose of Largactil—I spent an anxious few hours after one of my patients collapsed having been given a mere 25 mg of Largactil by injection. Noradrenaline, given in an intravenous drip, counteracts the effect of the Largactil where positioning of the patient does not suffice to keep the patient conscious, but I have never had to use it.

4. Skin reactions, including 'photosensitivity' (whereby patients on chlorpromazine easily develop severe sunburn) drug rashes, and dermatitis in some of those who handle chlorpromazine and become sensitive to it. The liquid forms of chlorpromazine are especially liable to cause sensitivity when the skin is exposed to them, and should therefore be handled with caution.

5. Obesity, due to stimulation of the appetite.

6. Depression (see p. 107).

7. Much less common than the above are jaundice (which is not serious if the drug is stopped straight away), fits (in those who are predisposed), depletion of the white blood cells, and pigmentation of the retina, a rare complication of thioridazine therapy which causes blindness.

Minor tranquillisers

For many years the drugs most widely used in the treatment of anxiety were barbiturates—phenobarbitone or sodium amytal, 30 to 60 mg two or three times a day. Now, however, the benzodiazepines are prescribed far more often, for though five times as costly and probably no more effective they are far safer. They have an action on the brain itself, calming anxiety, and on the nervous pathways to the muscles, thus relieving muscular tension.

The following are used mainly by day:

Chlordiazepoxide (Librium) was the first to be introduced, in 1960, and is given in a dosage of 5–20 mg three times a day by mouth.

Diazepam (Valium) 2–10 mg three times a day by mouth, or 10 mg by injection, has a particularly strong muscle-relaxing action.

Oxazepam (Serenid) 10–30 mg three times a day, by mouth.

Lorazepam (Ativa), probably the strongest of the group, is given in a dosage of 1–2·5 mg three times a day by mouth. Other 'azepams' are clorazepam (Tranxene) which, though usually given once in the 24 hours and at night, is meant to act during the day, clobazam (Frisium) and medazepam (Nobrium). Within the same group are several hypnotics, given at night to induce sleep—nitrazepam, flurazepam, temazepam, triazolam (see below).

Side-effects are unusual and not serious. They include drowsiness, rashes, and very rarely indeed, unsteadiness and muscular spasm. Physical dependency has been described, with a need to increase the dosage to get the same effect, and withdrawal symptoms when the drug is suddenly stopped, chiefly agitation, aching and trembling, are not uncommon, but avoidable if the dose is reduced very gradually.

The minor tranquillisers do relieve anxiety. They are an indifferent substitute for understanding and imparting insight into the difficulties in relationships which are so often the basis of the anxiety, but useful adjuncts to support and psychotherapy. They are not of course antidepressives, and are liable to misuse when the depressive basis of an apparent anxiety state is not recognised.

Before leaving the tranquillisers and passing to the antidepressives, mention must be made of chlormethiazole (Heminevrin), which does not belong either to the major or the minor category, but has a useful place in the management of acute confusional states. 0·5–1 g is given up to three times a day by mouth. Heminevrin is mainly used when chlorpromazine or haloperidol are not producing the desired effect. It should not be given at the same time as there drugs as it increases their activity to an extent said to be dangerous.

The antidepressives
Antidepressives are not stimulants. They have no effect on the normal mood, unlike the amphetamines (e.g. Dexedrine and 'purple hearts') which are 'pep pills' and are taken (usually these days illegally) for 'kicks', to produce energy and zest. Before the introduction of the first antidepressive in 1959 the amphetamines were quite widely used in the treatment of depression, and were of some value in lifting the mood of the moderately depressed for a little while. However, they tend to be habit-forming, and their effect in relieving depressive illness is much inferior to the antidepressives.

There are two groups of antidepressives: the *tricyclics* and the *monoamine oxidase inhibitors* (MAOIs for short). One of the latter groups, iproniazid (Marsilid—now no longer in use) was the first antidepressive to be discovered—by serendipity (a happy accident). It is structurally similar to isoniazid, which is an important antituberculous drug. Iproniazid, introduced for the treatment of tuberculosis, was found to lift the mood of depressed patients suffering from that disease, and was then noted to be useful for depressed patients in general. The tricyclics have a somewhat similar structure to the phenothiazines. The first tricyclic was imipramine (Tofranil), and this and amitriptyline (Tryptizol) are still the most widely used antidepressives.

Antidepressives take at least one week, usually two and sometimes three or more to act. As side-effects develop much earlier, as a rule, than benefit, careful explanation is needed to ensure that the patient takes them for long enough. They probably relieve rather than cure the depression, so must be taken for at least three months, and often for longer, until the underlying depression has remitted. They are not in the least habit-forming.

Tricyclics
These are regarded as the safer antidepressives (although side-effects are pretty common) and are therefore most often prescribed.

Imipramine given in a dose of 25–75 mg three times a day by mouth is effective but slow—one can wait for results as long as three weeks after reaching the highest dose. Sometimes, for quicker effect, it is given by injection (25 mg three times a day).

Amitriptyline, given in a dosage of 25–50 mg three times a day by mouth, is more sedative, and appears to act a little more quickly. It may also be given in a single dose of 50–100 mg at night which is useful for elderly depressives who do not take tablets very reliably (though it is often hard for them to understand that they are still taking an antidepressive, and not a sleeping tablet).

The preparation, Lentizol, need only be given once daily (usually at night): a 50 mg capsule is equivalent to 25 mg of Tryptizol given three times in a day.

Trimipramine (Surmontil), the most sedative antidepressive, is given in a single dose of 25–100 mg by mouth at night. This enhances the effect of any sleeping tablet and sometimes eliminates the need for one.

Protriptyline (Concordin) is the least sedative tricyclic. Given in a dose of 5–20 mg three times a day by mouth, it often acts within 7 to 10 days, and is of particular value for the retarded, apathetic depressive. Anxious and agitated patients, on the other hand, may be made worse.

Dothiepin (Prothiaden), 25–50 mg three times a day or 50–150 mg at night, has a lower incidence of side effects than any of the above, and acts usually within two weeks. It is probably the most generally useful drug for the treatment of depression in the elderly.

Clomipramine (Anafranil), 25–50 mg three times a day by mouth or 50–150 mg at night by mouth, or occasionally in a daily intravenous dose of 25 mg diluted in 500 ml. water and administered as a drip is stronger than any of the foregoing and more likely to produce anticholinergic side effects (see below). It is likely to be used for severe depression when one of the other tricyclics has failed.

Side-effects

1. All tricyclics cause some dryness of the mouth. By a similar mechanism, constipation, difficulty in passing water, and blurring of vision and sweating are occasionally produced. Much more rarely there is impotence and actual paralysis of the bowel.

2. Drowsiness is especially associated with the use of amitryptyline and trimipramine, while all may cause weight gain.

3. All are liable to affect the conduction of nerve impulses within the heart. This is more obvious on the electrocardiogram than clinically (unless a frank overdose has been taken) but these drugs should be used with caution in those with a history of cardiac disease, especially recent myocardial infarction (coronary thrombosis) or cardiac irregularity. That said, it is rare indeed, even in a psychogeriatric practice, to feel unable to use a tricyclic for these reasons where one is needed, or to find that cardiac complications arise from so doing.

4. Tremor, shakiness and unsteadiness of gait are occasional.

5. Fits are sometimes induced in the predisposed.

6. Agitation may be exacerbated by by imipramine, protryptyline and clomipramine. Delirium is a rare development, in patients of all ages. Schizophrenia is sometimes released or aggravated in the predisposed.

7. Tricyclics oppose the action of certain drugs given for high blood pressure (bethanidine, guanethidine), potentiate noradrenaline (sometimes used in local anaesthetics) and are themselves potentiated by babiturates. Most troublesome side-effects tend to lessen with continuing use of the drug.

MAOIs

Three are in common use:

Tranylcypromine (Parnate) 10–20 mg two or three times a day by mouth, is the most powerful and the least safe. Many patients experience a stimulating effect within two or three days, and this is followed by a true antidepressive action in one or two weeks. Because of this stimulation the last daily dose should not be taken much later than 2 p.m. or there will be difficulty in getting off to sleep. Commonly the drug is combined with a small tranquillising dose of trifluoperazine (1 mg with 10 mg of the antidepressive) as Parstelin; very occasionally the tranquilliser produces side-effects — muscular spasms. *Phenelzine* (Nardil), 15–30 mg three times a day by mouth, is the most widely used. *Isocarboxiazid* (Marplan), 10–20 mg three times a day by mouth, is the weakest and safest. Its main use is in combination with amitriptyline or dothiepin trimipramine in some cases of depression which fail to respond to either group of antidepressives alone.

Side-effects are far fewer than from the tricyclics. A drop in blood pressure, causing faintness, is the most common.

The main dangers are from the interaction with certain foods and other drugs. A *rise in blood pressure*, causing at the least a very unpleasant ache at the back of the head, and at the worst death from brain haemorrhage, can be produced by the drugs amphetamine and ephedrine and foods rich in the amino-acid tyramine (i.e. cheese, yeast extracts and pickled herrings). The action of some other drugs may be enhanced or potentiated because MAOIs interfere with the mechanisms (especially those in the liver) which normally break them down. Consequently patients on MAOIs need to be warned about the dangerous foods, and to avoid taking other drugs unless assured by a doctor or chemist that they are safe. A card setting out these precautions is usually issued with the first prescription. Even so, and although dangerous reactions are in practice rare, the drugs should not be given lightly, especially to those who are too dim, muddled or feckless to take them responsibly.

Tricyclics are the antidepressives of first choice for both severe and milder depression. They are safer than the MAOIs, and often effective. Also, if it proves necessary to switch to an MAOI after all, the change can be made within a day or two of stopping the tricyclic, which is quickly eliminated from the body, whereas there should be an interval of three weeks between stopping an MAOI and starting a tricyclic.

However, for the anxious, hypochondriacal, neurotic minor depressive, whose symptoms vary from day to day, who feels more miserable towards evening, who is more irritable than guilty, and who has difficulty in getting to sleep, MAOIs are rather more likely to help. They also have a place in the treatment of some resistant cases of the more typical depressive illnesses.

Tricyclics are among the drugs with which the MAOIs should not normally be combined, but certain mixture, i.e. isocarboxiazid with amitriptyline, phenelzine with trimipramine, are relatively safe and sometimes of value where depression is otherwise intractable.

The new antidepressives

There is a constant quest for the perfect antidepressive, swift in action, highly effective, with few or no side-effects, and very safe. It hasn't been found yet.

Contenders for the title are usually competing with the tricyclics rather than the MAOIs, and aim in particular to act more quickly and with less by way of anticholinergic side-effects and less potential danger to the heart. Some, like *maprotiline* (Ludiomil) are not all that disimilar from the tricyclics in their chemical structure, while others, such as *tradozone* (Molipaxin) are very different. *Viloxazine* (Vivalan) has proved too often nauseating to be widely used. Of the tetracyclics, *mianserine* (Bolvidon) 60–120 mg daily may relieve depression in less than a fortnight. Drowsiness may occur at a lower dosage.

Another tetracyclic, *nomifensine* (Merital), 50–200 mg daily usually given in divided doses, potentiates dopamine and might therefore be the antidepressive of choice in patients also suffering from Parkinsonism. The more different the chemical formula of the drug is from the tricyclics the greater, perhaps, the chance that it will work in cases of resistant depression. As yet, however, while these new antidepressives are in various ways a little safer than the older, none has been shown to be more effective and the more established drugs retain the principal place in the treatment of depression.

Other drugs used for depression

Certain of the drugs listed in the formulary as stimulants of the central nervous system may be preferred to the antidepressives in frail debilitated elderly patients who are weary, demoralised and physically unwell. In these one way may well want a quick 'pick me up' without side effects. The 'tonic', which so many patients seek, can hardly be said to exit, but substances such as *pemoline* (Kethamed) 20–40 mg once or twice a day, *fencamfamin* (plus a few vitamins—Reactivan) one or two tablets a day and *methylphenidate* (Ritalin) 10–20 mg once or twice a day may raise spirits and alertness a little, just as may a good strong cup of tea or coffee.

Amphetamine belongs in this group and although its use in the treatment of depression must be very limited indeed (for the reasons given on p. 152) it has in my opinion a small place for depressed demented subjects who seem to tolerate the conventional antidepressives ill and to get little benefit from them (see p. 59).

Flupenthixol (Fluanxol) has already been mentioned. 0·5–1 mg twice a day by mouth (not towards evening, or troublesome wake-

fulness may ensue) seem to benefit many mild to moderate depressives more quickly than do the tricyclics, with fewer side-effects.

L. *tryptophan* (Pacitron, or, with added vitamins, Optimax),
1 gm. three times a day is supposed to help in the treatment of
depression by being the precursor (forerunner) of one of the
neurotransmitters presumed to be depleted in the synapses of the
brain in that disorder. It rarely achieves much when prescribed
alone, but sometimes potentiates MAOIs and is therefore of occasional value in the treatment of resistant (or refractory) depression.
However the tablets are on the large side! A full account of *Lithium
carbonate* has already been given (p. 98). Preparations available include Camcolit 250 or 400 mg tablets, Priabil 400 mg tablets, Phasal 300 mg tablets and Liskonum 450 mg tablets, the latter three are
all slow relse preparations which aim to reduce frequency of dosage
to as little as once a day. Dosage should achieve a blood level of
$0·6-1.2$ mEq/1. Side effects include a fine tremor, thirst, and
weight gain; toxicity is suggested by diarrhoea, vomiting and confusion, and these symptoms indicate that the drug should be stopped at once and the lithium level checked. Lithium has a place in
the treatment of frequently recurrent and incapacitating bipolar or
even unipolar depression, unless severe cardiac or renal disease
makes it use too risky.

Hypnotics

A hypnotic is a drug given to induce *sleep*. A sedative is a smaller
dose of a similar drug given to calm the anxious or disturbed.

Hypnotics are useful in the whole range of psychiatric disorders,
where sleep is impaired, but, as has been indicated several times in
earlier chapters, are easily abused. It is disconcerting that the elderly are the greatest users of hypnotics. Many of those must be abusers,
who take the drugs because they are bored, depressed, in pain
or so much in the habit of sleeping for seven hours at night that
they do not realise that they can manage just as well in later life
with five. Where possible, it is always preferable to deal with the
cause of sleeplessness, including also cold, noise, and other discomfort and lack of exercise, rather than have recourse to a sleeping
tablet. An analgesic (pain-relieving drug) such as aspirin or para-
cetamol, or a sedative antidepressant, such as trimipramine (Surmontil) may on occasion be more appropriate. A warm milk drink
before retiring, an active day, a comfortable bed with sufficient
bedclothes, a properly heated room, quiet, and relief of unnecessary anxiety all help to keep the use of hypnotics down. In institutions, avoidance of measures which are designed to give the night

staff a quiet time, rather than truly to give the patients or residents essential sleep, has a similar effect. I refer to practices such as putting everyone to bed early and the routine prescribing of hypnotics for all.

Abuse of hypnotics leads to habituation, dependency, intoxication, confusion, falls, incontinence and bedsores. However, for the delirious or manic patient who is not getting enough rest, the severe depressive who wakes early in the moring feeling at his lowest, the anxious or less seriously depressed patient who cannot get to sleep and the restless demented patient who is up in the small hours disturbing others and not knowing what time it is, hypnotics have an important place.

Those in common use are the benzodiazepines, chloral derivatives and chlormathiazole, while there are still many regular users of barbiturates and alcohol.

Benzodiazepine hypnotics are popular because they are safe and pretty effective, which is not to say that they are without side-effects, the most troublesome of which is drowsiness the next morning. It may not be properly appreciated by the patient's attendants that sleepiness, unsteadiness and a lack of alertness at the beginning of the day are not just due to the infirmity of age but are drug induced.

Nitrazepam (Mogadon) 5–10 mg is probably the most widely prescribed hypnotic at all ages; it induces sleep by reducing wakefulness, and is undoubtedly useful, but may not fully eliminated from the body within 24 hours and so may cause a hangover next day and, if given regularly, may accumulate so that the taker is continuously under its influence. These effects are still more marked in the next more commonly prescribed benzodiazepine hynpotic *flurazepam* (Dalmane) which should therefore, in my opinion, never be given to the elderly.

Much shorter in their length of action, and therefore especially suitable for those whose difficulty is in falling asleep, are *triazolam* (Halcion) 0·125–0·25 mg nocte and *temazepam* (Euphynos, Normison) 10–30 mg.

Chloral hydrate 1–2g, well diluted, has for many years been the hypnotic of choice for the elderly, though its supremacy is now challenged by nitrazepam. The draught is bitter, but most old people take it very well. It is safe and effective. These days, however, it is more often given as a tablet, e.g. *dichloralphenazone* (Welldorm) 650 mg, or *triclofos* (Tricloryl) 500 mg, one to four tablets at night.

Chlormethiazole (Heminevrin) 500–1000 mg is a hypnotic chemically unlike the foregoing with a relatively short action, which may work where the others do not and is most unlikely to cause a hangover, though sometimes it has the odd side-effect of inducing sneezing.

Barbiturates

Barbiturates, e.g. amylobarbitone sodium (Sodium Amytal) 200–400 mg, quinalbarbitone sodium (Seconal) 100 mg should by now be obselete, because although cheap and very effective they may produce acute confusional states in old people and there are extra changes of dependency and sometimes fatal overdosage. Many of the elderly still take them, understandably, because they have long done so (i.e. they are habituated), but they should never be prescribed where they have not been given previously.

Alcohol, the traditional 'nightcap', is effective and agreeable, but rarely available on a NHS prescription. A nightly whisky is beyond the resources of most pensioners, and anyway, the immediate hypnotic effect is rather offset by the subsequent tendency to promote urination.

PHYSICAL TREATMENTS

Electroplexy

The discovery of the value of convulsive therapy in psychiatry is another example of serendipity. The erroneous clinical observation that epileptics are less susceptible than others to schizophrenia (in fact they are more so) led to attempts artificially (by chemical means, e.g. injection of camphor) to induce fits in schizophrenics. This was found to be effective in mute and withdrawn patients (i.e. suffering the catatonic form of schizophrenia) and later to be most beneficial of all not to schizophrenics, but to the severely depressed. The Italians Cerletti and Bini then elaborated an electrical means of inducing fits, more certain and less unpleasant than using drugs for the purpose, and thus in 1938 ECT came into being. It was rapidly adopted in mental hospitals all over the world, and proved by far the most dramatic and effective treatment so far available to psychiatry; and as far as the treatment of severe depression goes, it still is.

ECT used to be given 'straight', to fully conscious patients, a painless procedure of which the patient had no subsequent memory, but causing a vigorous convulsion which occasionally led to wrenched muscles and fractures. Now the fit is 'modified' by the use of a short-acting anaesthetic to put the patient to sleep, and a muscle-relaxant which reduces the convulsion to the merest twitching of the muscles, without any lessening of benefit though with a very slight increase in the risk to life.

The use of ECT in depression has been fully described on pages 81–82. I will merely reiterate here that for the severely depressed patient who is not responding to antidepressives, is eating and drinking too little and is becoming suicidal, its use is essential. Those who decry it in the elderly are sentimental and ill-informed. ECT for suitable patients not only relieves intolerable anguish, but saves life. A measure of scepticism towards psychiatry and psychiatrists, especially within the profession itself, is healthy. They are not omnipotent gurus, and rarely want to be regarded as such. Sometimes their clinical skills have been prostituted to politcal ends in totalitarian states. However ECT is not a brain washing technique in the free world, but a reputable and reliable remedy for one of the very worst forms of human suffering. For some years now psychiatrists convinced of the value of the treatment have been reluctant on ethical grounds to subject it to the scientific test of a double blind trial (Kendell, 1981). This means giving some patients the anaesthetic followed by the treatment while others have the anaesthetic only, and neither they nor those who assess them are supposed to know to which group they belong. Lately, however, some psychiatrists have bowed to public disquiet and overcome the problem of finding enough suitable subjects able to give informed consent to such an experiment. For example, West (1981) did a double blind cross-over (meaning that those who got the anaesthetic only at first were eventually given ECT if they still needed it) trial on 22 subjects and found the results of the treatment significantly better than those of the placebo at every point.

Psychosurgery
The first *leucotomy* was performed by Egas Moniz in 1935. This operation, by cutting the fibres between the nerve cells on the surface of the front of the brain and those in the thalamus, in the middle of the brain, can greatly reduce emotional tension. The early operations, though, by cutting a great many fibres, produced a most undersirable personality change, towards callous selfishness; fits were another complication. Over the years psychosurgery has become more precise and refined, and by cutting as few fibres as possible, though still able to relieve tension, the incidence of complications has been much reduced. Patients are far more carefully selected than in the 1930s and 1940s, and there is a much wider

range of effective and less final alternative treatments now, so that psychosurgery has become something of a rarity; indeed, in many centres it is regarded as obsolete.

This is by no means altogether a good thing, for there is a small but very important minority of patients suffering chronic severe tension, due to agitated depression, obsessional-compulsive neurosis or anxiety state, their lives completely crippled by their affliction, who can obtain from leucotomy lasting relief which no other form of treatment can match. To consign such patients to lasting misery in the long-stay wards of a mental hospital for the sake of the principle that the personality is sacred and that psychosurgery is immoral, is misguided idealism.

Among the elderly the prevalence of chronic tension states is relatively high, and psychosurgery can be of substantial benefit. The personality established over so many years is not greatly affected by the operation. After surgery there may be a period of confusion, and intensive rehabilitation over weeks or months is needed to reap the greatest benefit.

Probably the operation of choice for the elderly is that of stereotactic tractotomy. The use of this in the treatment of chronic depressive illness has been described on pages 84–85.

REFERENCES

Kendell R E 1981 The present status of electroconvulsive therapy. Brit J Psychiat 139: 265.
West E D 1981 Electric convulsion therapy in depression: a double-blind controlled trial. Brit Med J 1: 355

15

Psychological therapies

PSYCHOTHERAPY

Psychotherapy is based upon a *dynamic* view of psychiatric (and some physical) illnesses. The word 'dynamic' suggests drive and movement, but where psychiatric symptoms arise *conflict* has led to a stalemate. The conflict may be internal e.g. between the drive to assert oneself as a man and the drive to obtain parental approval by continuing to be a good obedient boy, or external, with someone to whom one is very close but with whom one cannot agree. The ultimate object of psychotheraphy is by resolving conflict to relieve symptoms and help the personality (ego) to function more effectively. This is achieved through the words exchanged by the patient and the therapist and the relationship which forms between them. Dynamic psychiatry recognises the tremendous importance of disturbed *relationships*, past and present, in the development of illness and psychotherapy seeks to improve these relationships by counselling, support and the use of transference—whereby the patient reacts to the therapist as if he were a key figure (such as parent, brother, child, spouse) from the past.

Despite the importance of organic factors, such as ageing and brain disease, in psychogeriatrics, dynamic considerations do not dwindle away in patients who have reached the age of 65, but frequently determine when and how an illness develops, and when it is brought to the attention of others. As has already been described in Chapter 2, the senium is period of loss and growing dependency, with which many old people cannot cope. In Chapter 6, it has been pointed out that the fifth of demented patients cared for in institutions are not simply those most disturbed and incapacitated, but also the most isolated and the least liked. The chapters on depression, neurosis, and personality and behaviour disorder have described how disturbed relationships contribute to, as well as arise from these conditions.

I once looked through my records of 20 successive old people whom I had been asked to see at home. They may be briefly summarised as follows:

1. Marital crisis—yet again—between a quaint couple who label each other mentally ill whenever tension between them becomes too high.

2. Depressive illness, masquerading as loneliness (Mrs Jacobs, p. 79).

3. A lady who appears sometimes paranoid, sometimes depressed, but never divulges enough for a clear formulation to be made. She had become much more withdrawn and suspicious while the son with whom she lives had been at home on holiday.

4. A subnormal woman with chronic schizophrenia, maintained by Modecate injections and the Salvation Army, whose GP had become worried about her for reasons which never became very clear.

5. A psychiatrically normal old lady presented as 'scapegoat' during a family crisis: her daughter-in-law, with whom she lived, had advanced cancer, and the daughter who lived nearby was reluctan to take over the old lady's care.

6. An old lady frightened by early dementia and reacting like an insecure child, clinging to her daughter, abusing her and feeling miserable.

7. A chronic neurotic depressive who dominates her unmarried daughter and whose symptoms are exacerbated when the daughter seems to be settling into a job.

8. A previously demented old lady, in an old people's home, now suffering from a stroke and apparently referred to me because of dissatisfaction with the failure of the casualty department of the general hospital to admit her.

9. Mild agitated depression in the wife of a neglectful husband, very dependent on her children, who were apparently being punished for having for the first time in their lives taken a holiday without her.

10. An almost identical lady who, again, I thought was registering 'holiday protest'. I was wrong; she turned out to have cancer of the stomach and died three months later.

11. A spirited old man, suffering from variable confusion and occasionally aggressive because of cerebral atherosclerosis, long resident in a Salvation Army eventide home but found difficult by new staff.

12. Another resident of the same home, paranoid, depressed, brain-damaged and personality-disordered, but probably mainly reacting to the staff change.

13. An elderly Jewess, psychiatrically normall but living too limited a life since her stroke and getting on the nerves of her single, middle-age daughter who lived with her.

14. A demented old man, living alone but regularly seen to by his daughter, living nearby, whose husband was protesting that she was spending too much time out of the house and with the old man: A problem of her divided loyalties.

15. Another marital problem, between a stubborn old 90-year-old and his wife of 88 who complained that he was violent towards her and more than once involved the police in their rows. I could find no evidence that either was mentally ill.

16. A manipulative chronic invalid, with a history of physical and psychiatric problems stretching back over years, and her collusive, guilty, dominated husband, asking yet again if anything could be done and, as usual, raising objections to every solution offered.

17. A demented old lady who kept quarrelling with her uncomprehending husband and was too vigorously supported by their subnormal daughter, who had been taken to court for her assaults on the old man.

18. A delirious episode, quite over by the time I visited, in an apparently fit elderly woman living alone who had been upset not to be taken by her son on holiday, but had also recently been in hospital with pneumonia and heart failure. The diagnosis here (as not infrequently) was GOK—God Only Knows!

19. A demented old man who had fathered 27 children by his two wives. Neighbours had complained of the smell of his incontinence, and his dull, demoralised wife (who had borne 17 of the children) was under some pressure to 'get him away'.

20. Mania in a chronic manic-depressive living in an old people's home.

These 20 cases seem to be pretty typical of those referred to my psychogeriatric service. It will be seen that dynamic factors were of far more importance than the onset of a clear-cut psychiatric illness in determining referral. Indeed, a precise psychiatric diagnosis was made in less than half, whereas, disturbed relationships were of major importance in almost three-quarters.

Goldfarb (1965) explains that patients, especially those referred to hospitals and homes, react badly to the social and biological stresses of ageing which, indeed, relatively few people handle well. The patient's symptoms, or the behaviour complained of by others, often arise from a decline in self-esteem and self-confidence. There is a lack of motivation, of a sense of purpose, after the loss of valued people, and there is no longer the ability to act in the ways thought necessary to bind others in supportive relationships. Believing himself to be very weak, the old person makes another, whom he believes to be strong, a quasi-parent figure. He then searches for and tries to win and hold such a person. Dependent behaviour of this sort is in fact a continuation of a dependent way of life, but previously less evident as such. For example, serviceable behaviour to others—being masculine and dependable, feminine and caring, motherly and supportive, may all be ways of gaining strength from others by making them rely on oneself; these techniques are no longer available to the frail, infirm old person.

In the collusive partnership so often encountered in psychogeriatrics—child/parent, husband/wife—one is seen by the other as strong, but each is in fact intensely dependent on the other. The 'strong' partner preserves an illusion of mastery through the 'weaker's' reliance on him. The husband who finds his raison d'être after retirement in caring for a sick wife is seriously threatened when she no longer looks solely to him, but turns to doctors. He has then to interfere with therapy in order to stay 'one up'—which means seeing to it that she remains 'one down'.

The physical treatments described in the previous chapter have a very important place, especially where there is serious, sustained disturbance of mood, or paranoia, for without them it may not be possible to communicate properly, (while they also symbolise the potency which the patient seeks from the therapist); however they are not sufficient for the intensely anxious and dependent. Such patients make incomplete recoveries, relapse speedily or develop a new picture of suffering to present to another agency. Environmental manipulation is frequently required to offset the losses which appear to have turned the person into a patient—day care, rehousing, enlistment of the various community services (see Ch. 16). However these too will not suffice for those who want neither pills, nor a change of scene, but *people*. With such patients the therapist tries to establish a supportive relationship which will meet the dependency needs without the therapist's feeling taken over altogether, or the patient's being turned into a child. *Supportive* psychotherapy is usually an involvement for life (though the life is not always all that long).

Goldfarb observes that the goal of psychotherapy is to raise the patient's self-esteem. The more affectionate are content with the gratification that someone good and powerful seems to care for them. Others derive satisfaction from the idea that by their own wit, wisdom, cunning, subtlety and cleverness they are 'having' the therapist as a protective ally; not only do they enlist his strength on their behalf but there is the triumph of achievement in having 'caught' him.

Wayne (1952), another psychotherapist with experience of the elderly, states that the therapist's approach may be genuinely warm and friendly, and that there is a place for pleasant personal remarks which are generally taboo to younger patients. At the same time, confrontation with negative reactions to the therapist, like jealousy, patronising, plaintiveness and exaggeration of symptoms, is appropriate. Treatment should be tailed off, rather than officially concluded.

I find such confrontations essential if I am to feel at ease as a supporter, and I am satisfied that they do nothing but good provided that the patient understands that 'having things out' is not a prelude to rejection. It is also a useful technique, when the recitation of symptoms has become tedious and repetitive, to move away to a consideration of the patient as a person with an interesting store of reminiscences to offset the dullness of the present limited existence (see Mr Gordon, p. 116).

Butler (1968) advocates a 'life review' which helps the elderly patient to function by gaining strength from past experience of survival and adaptation.

For some, group support is the best means of meeting dependency needs. It is less fraught than intense involvement with an individual, and less likely to lead to regression. *Group therapy*, however, presents some special difficulties with the elderly. Many patients are too deaf to hear anything delivered at less than a bellow, and some are too confused to know that they are in a group at all. This is eliminated by selection of outpatient groups, but not in wards run along 'therapeutic community' lines, where every patient is entitled to a seat in the group (p. 147). Somnolence, which may be interpreted as 'resistance' but may well at times be physiological, has also to be reckoned with. Avoidance of meeting after heavy meals; the use of hard, straight-backed chairs which allow a tighter circle than armchairs and are more difficult to sleep in; and well-ventilated rooms, with as few distractions as possible and a minimum of extraneous noise, all help to keep everybody awake and able to hear. There is, however, a strong tendency to ignore the other members of the group and speak only to the staff—a resistance which is far more difficult to overcome. To encourage interest in the others it may be a good idea for every meeting to start with every member of the group identifying himself or herself, to introduce newcomers, to discuss those who have gone (the dead as well as the quick) and, in the ward situation, those who are giving concern by their disturbed or sick behaviour. The recognition that old people are worth listening to, and talking with, the democratic arrangement whereby all, staff and patients, sit together in a circle, and the opportunity to discover that it can be safe to express grievances directly, as protest, rather than through helplessness, are all valuable benefits of group therapy in psychogeriatrics, however silent or disconnected the meetings may often appear to be. A further practical point: meetings should not run longer than half an hour—this is as much as the patients can cope with, or most staff stand.

Finally, not all domestic tensions arise from dependency or collusion. Other problems include the strain of married life after retirement, where couples who no longer like each other very much are forced into each other's company all day (p. 14). Two forms of neglect are suggested by literature. The first is the 'King Lear' situation, where care for the old person is shared in turn by less and less devoted children. The second is the 'Oedipal' situation when a single child living with both parents forms an alliance with one to the exclusion of the other, usually bachelor son with mother, father being left out in the cold (see Mr Gordon, p. 116). The distress, anger, anxiety and guilt felt by families frequently require consideration in their own right (see Ch. 18). Consequently there is a need for *marital therapy*, directed towards the expression of resentment in a way which the couple do not find totally destructive, and *family therapy*, which views the problem as one shared by the whole family which, rather than any individual, 'the patient', in psychogeriatric psychotherapy.

BEHAVIOUR THERAPY

As Freud must be regarded as the father of psychotherapy, his Russian near contemporary Pavlov was the prime source of behaviour therapy. Pavlov showed that the reflex salivation of dogs at the smell of food was also induced by the sound of a bell which they had learnt to precede the giving of the food, and called this 'conditioning'. The idea that conditioning is the basis of neurotic symptoms and behaviour disorders is fundamental to behaviour therapy: these are, as it were, bad habits which have been learnt, and may be unlearnt. The idea of a dynamic unconscious is irrelevant to behavioural psychology: never mind where the problem arose, the task is to remove it. The techniques are derived from *learning theory* and include:

1. *Systematic desensitization* whereby the patient gradually learns

not to panic when faced with a previously feared object or situation, e.g. cats or supermarkets.

2. *Flooding* which is a 'diving in at the deep end' approach to the same sort of problem.

3. *Conditioned aversion*, whereby a desired but destructive form of behaviour is given very unpleasant associations, e.g. vomiting with drink for alcoholics, an electric shock with sexual arousal for certain forms of sexual deviation.

4. *Operant conditioning*, a system of consistent rewards and disincentives which selectively reinforce good behaviour and not 'bad'. The 'habit training' and 'token economy' used especially in the social rehabilitation of chronic schizophrenia and subnormal subjects are really aspects of operant conditioning: the 'tokens' which reward 'good behaviour' can be used to purchase comforts or privileges.

Other techniques less wholly based upon learning theory include modelling, rôle play, and social skills training. In *modelling* identification with an other or others helps the subject to take the same risks; in *rôle play* situations which arouse incapacitating anxiety can be acted, e.g. an old lady nervous about going to the post office; *social skills* training helps shy, gauche inhibited people to cope with the basic social situations, like making conversation, which most of us take for granted.

All these techniques, to which may be added the reality orientation therapy and reminiscence aids (p. 55) for the demented, may be applicable to elderly patients: we are rapidly learning that old people can learn. A behavioural psychologist is now a much needed member of the psychogeriatric team, not only to treat patients directly but to teach others how to do so.

Pages 88 and 129 discuss further the use of operant conditioning, in particular in the treatment of behaviour disorder associated with depression and in its own right.

REFERENCES

Butler R N 1968 Towards a psychiatry of the life cycle: implications of sociopsychologic studies of the ageing process for the psychotherapeutic selection. In: Simon A, Epstein L J (eds) Ageing and modern society. Psychiatric research reports of the American Psychiatric Association, Washington DC
Goldfarb A 1965 The recognition and therapeutic use of the patient's search for aid. In: Psychiatric disorders in the aged. WPA Symposium. Geigy, Manchester
Wayne G J 1952 Psychotherapy in senescence. Amer West Med & Surg 6: 88

16

Social therapy and rehabilitation

This chapter is concerned with those social measures which enable an old person to live as full and independent a life as possible, and with the principles and techniques by which a patient is assisted to make the most of residual abilities.

Social therapy includes the personal supportive services made available to the elderly at home; adjustments to accommodation; and day care.

SUPPORTIVE SERVICES

In England and Wales these are now largely the responsibility of the Director of Social Services employed by the local authority. Departments of social services were massively reorganised a few years ago (Seebohm, 1978) and in many areas there is a considerable gap between need and the service provided; this is because of attitudes as well as limited resources. As yet most departments appear to meet very obvious needs on an ad hoc basis, and in a more practical (but still frequently inadequate) than imaginative way. For example, a problem of self-neglect is more likely to be dealt with by the provision of a home help or Meals on Wheels, or placement on the lengthy waiting list for a residential home, than by giving the old person regular *personal* support. Case finding and preventive work are largely unknown. *Social workers* are now 'generic', i.e. instead of specialising in certain areas such as child care or mental health they bring their skills to bear on the whole range of social problems referred to the Social Services Department. This is fine in principle, and may eventually become so in practice, but as yet many social workers are confronted with situations which they lack the training, experience or sometimes even the inclination to cope with. To the outsider the system of allocating cases, which seems to depend upon the willingness of one of the team to become involved, is arbitrary and inefficient. There may be delays of weeks before it is decided who, if anyone, will take on Mrs Green who was referred for support on her discharge from hospital. The argument that Mrs Green should not have been discharged until it was known who would be dealing with her takes no account of the pressures on the hospital and medical services generally to work at a pace which too few social services departments seem ready to match. Only a minority of social workers appear to have much interest in working with the elderly (in this respect they are much like doctors and nurses), and the remainder by avoiding such clients never develop the knowledge or expertise which would make them effective. There is a significant regrettable tendency for the elderly to be left to untrained social workers. There is far too little casework in depth with the elderly and their families, and far too much so-called support seems designed to reassure the worker that he need not call very often or for very long. The attitude that social work with old people means no more than finding a home, seeing to the rent or looking after the budgie is far too prevalent.

These may sound harsh words from a doctor, but I have been equally critical in this book of some of my colleagues and of the hospital services they provide, and my intention is not destructive but to point out glaring inadequacies so that they may be remedied. The full potential of the community social worker in providing moral as well as practical support has yet to be realised. The impact of a strike of social workers in Britain, in some places lasting as long as a year, on the welfare of the elderly, was small; disconcertingly so, in a way!

An example of less than sensitive professional advice is provided by a contrary old Eurasian, stone deaf following typhoid but able to lip-read until cataracts caused his sight to fail, but then sensorily cut off and anyway, having lived most of his life in India, at sea in an alien culture. He had been happily married to a wife who waited on him hand and foot. After her death 14 years ago he lived with his eldest daughter in the Midlands, but somehow got on her nerves to such a degree that she became mentally ill and he went into a home. He failed to settle down, and prevailed upon his younger daughter to take him into her crowded slum home in the East End of London. However, he failed to settle there either, and wrote to the Social Services Department to be found another place in a home. He had expected to be sent back to the Midlands, but instead was placed in a pleasant, well run home very near his younger daughter. She was rehoused, in a better flat, still nearer the home, and when at Christmas, a year after he had left her, he beg-

ged her to take him back she did not hesitate to do so. She was
warned by the matron of the home that he might well change his
mind; in the home he had been solitary, demanding, changeable
and liable from time to time to take offence. Consequently he was
given a month's trial leave at home (which went very satisfactorily)
before his official discharge. When the last of his luggage came
from the home, however, he got into a state, claiming that it was
not his. His daughter insisted angrily that it was. The upshot was a
furious quarrel which ended in his storming out of the house with
the intention of finding his way back to the home. He blundered
across a busy main road, unable to hear the noise or to see properly
where he was going, and was rescued by a passing health visitor.
When she asked her social worker colleague what to do about this
problem she was simply advised, 'Cut off his fly-buttons!'

I was asked to see him later that day, back at his home, where I
met a gentle but almost impenetrably deaf old man who held an
omnipotent view of his world, believing that whatever he desired
should be brought speedily to pass. His daughter, a tall, spirited
woman, mother of three young children and working as a cleaner
in the evenings, showed an intriguing blend of intense filial devotion
and extreme exasperation. She clearly thought it her duty to make
a home for her father, and at the same time was irritated by him to
distraction. When I asked him questions, she repeated them to him
in a scream, her face apparently contorted with fury, in the ostensible effort of making him hear. In fact I found that I could communicate with him rather better on his own without having to raise
the roof. Here was a splendid, but so far missed, opportunity for
social casework. The 'answer' to the 'problem' was not to find the
old man another home, still less to subject him to the degrading
manoeuvre suggested (presumably tongue-in-cheek) by the social
worker, but to work with the whole local family, focusing on the
daughter's ambivalence, to help her fulfil her daughterly role as she
saw it and yet be able to tolerate her father and still function as
woman, mother of three young children and working as a cleaner in
tially as rewarding and challenging.

The social worker needs a mature understanding of the problems
of ageing for the individual and the family, knowledge of a vast
range of resources, the willingness and ability to liaise with a number of other agencies, and considerable flexibility, being ready to
deal with down-to-earth problems of pensions, front-door keys,
clothing and sanitation, at one moment, and complex emotional
situations at the next. Happily there are social workers in Britain
and elsewhere who well recognise all this and are keen not only to

see that all workers are better prepared to meet the needs of their older clients, but that some of them should specialise in this field (Plank, 1979)

The home help service is at present one of the main stays of geriatric and psychogeriatric care in the community. Home helps are superior domestics with a strong sense of service. They will cook, shop and collect pensions as well as clean, and being in closer contact with the old person who lives alone than anyone else, are the first to know, very often, when things are going seriously wrong. Under the direction of a supervisor they provide a first-class, responsible service. However, they are human, lack a professional training, can be insensitive and their goodwill is not infinite. I find that they are sometimes defeated by particularly cantankerous, ungrateful or filthy clients.

A useful modification of the home help service is the *Good Neighbours* scheme, whereby suitable neighbours are paid to help out old people in need.

Meals on Wheels have already been discussed (p. 17). There are problems in serving meals hot, appetising and for a variety of tastes, but these are generally tackled resourcefully. It is surprising that this remains so often a voluntary service, but the only real criticism is that in many areas it is not often enough available.

Other support is provided by the health services:

The *general practitioner* is a vital provider of personal service and coordinator of the efforts of others. If he is interested in his elderly patients none can do more for them. He is consulted as a matter of course about problems with a far wider range than the strictly medical, and he is available to his patients far more than anyone else. The single-handed GP who is a personal doctor to all his patients, on call at all times, however, is passing, and his place is being taken by the group practice and the health centre, which offset the disadvantages of less strictly individual care with better facilities and the services of district nurses and health visitors.

District and *community nurses* provide nursing in the home. The former are employed by the local authority, but may be attached to a group practice; they are general nurses (SRN) who give practical treatment—administering medicines, applying dressings, bathing (though in some areas this work has been taken over by special bathing attendants) and nursing patients through acute illnesses. Community nurses are psychiatrically trained, and employed either by the local authority or by the hospital to work within its catchment area. They are proving invaluable in providing at home the kind of treatment and support otherwise only available at the hospitals, thus enabling many patients to stay in the community. They follow up discharged patients (whom they will usually have met in the hospital) and supervise their medication; the administration of the long-acting fluphenazine injections (Modecate and Depixol—see p. 149) is but one of their functions. They are also called by the psychiatrist to deal with acute and crisis situations, and experience is suggesting that repeated visits over a relatively short period resolve many of these without there being any recourse to hospital admission. They also take direct referrals from other community workers, and are proving valuable advisers about the management of diverse tricky problems and giving guidance about who else should be consulted, where necessary, including of course, the psychiatrist.

Health visitors, usually attached to group practices, are generally trained nurses with special extra training in preventive and social medicine. As yet I feel that most have had too little to do with the elderly, and consequently, like social workers, they have rather a lot to learn about how effectively they can spot old people at risk and prevent the worst befalling them.

In every area in Britain an old people's welfare committee collects and disperses information about services for the elderly.

Volunteers come in a whole variety of forms, though there are rarely enough of them. The WRVS, who have already been mentioned as the suppliers of Meals on Wheels, also provide clothing and comforts. The Churches sometimes look after their own, and sometimes (like the Salvation Army) minister to all and sundry. *Age Concern* is an organisation which not only arranges local services, such as transport and socials, but also speaks eloquently on behalf of the elderly at large. *MIND* has taken a great interest in the older population of late, and has organised conferences and courses for all sorts of professionals and volunteers to improve and increase their knowledge of mental health problems in the elderly. Enthusiastic groups of young people (such as *Task Force* and sixth formers) can achieve a great deal, such as cleaning and decorating a house, in a very short time, though they do not so easily provide continuity of care. Volunteers who can be relied upon to visit regularly, who will act as sitters-in to enable the key supporter to have a break, and who are prepared to sit and listen, allowing the old person the 'blessing' of giving rather than simply receiving attentions, are particularly precious.

Mention in this section should also be made of the *Attendance Allowance* which offers some financial compensation to those who have to give so much time to a dependent relative that they cannot go out to work. The *Incontinent Laundry Service* is of immense value to those caring for intractably incontinent patients, who would otherwise have to wash out large quantities of foul linen daily; as yet the provision of this service by no means matches the need. *Cleansing and disinfestation* services are sometimes called in to homes which have reached a greater state of squalor than the home help can cope with. Rather surprisingly, in my experience, action is often laggardly once the old person has left her home, and there may be long delays before she can return. These are occasioned by the need as a rule to have her permission to enter the home and throw away refuse, and the desirability of having her actually in attendance when this is done: a typical psychogeriatric dilemma— knowing what is for the best, but respecting the old person's right to live as she likes.

ACCOMMODATION

Aspects of housing have already been considered; pages 16 and 144 have touched on housing policy, sheltered housing, and warden-supervision, while residential homes will be considered in more detail in Chapter 18. Here, adaptations to homes and boarding-out schemes will be briefly discussed.

Adaptations to render the existing home more habitable for the elderly occupant include normal repairs and safety measures— fixing loose boards, rugs and carpets, covering slippery surfaces, improving heat and lighting—and installing special aids to daily living (ADL) for the handicapped. Examples of useful aids are grab-rails in the lavatory and bathroom (if any), handrails in passages and stairways, and gadgets in the kitchen for those who lack the use of one arm. ADL are normally installed under the supervision of an occupational therapist. Grants for these adaptations may be obtained through the local authority where the handicap is 'permanent' and substantial, but frequently there is considerable delay when negotiations have to be made with a private landlord.

Boarding-out of the dependent elderly with suitably motivated landladies is an alternative to the use of residential homes which deserves more attention. The greatest successes have been with chronic (usually schizophrenic) patients from mental hospitals, but there is no reason why old people in the community who can no longer cope alone should not be similarly helped. Experience indicates that boarding-out schemes should be supervised by a social worker who takes a considerable interest in landlady and tenant, carefully preparing each for the other in the first place and following up regularly.

DAY CARE

This is available from day hospitals, centres, clubs and sheltered workshops.

Day hospitals provide medical and nursing treatment on a daily basis, usually, but not always, in premises which are part of a hospital for in-patients, to old people attending up to five or seven days a week, about half of whom generally require transport. The staff includes doctors, nurses, occupational therapists, physiotherapist, and social workers—in fact, the full psychogeriatric team—as well as the use of secretarial, domestic and kitchen workers. Patients may or may not have been in-patients previously, but all have suffered at least moderately severe psychiatric disorder, which either continues or seems likely to recur without the day hospital's support and supervision. Most are likely to be depressive, while demented patients are unlikely to account for even a half. Only demented patients whole condition is but slowly progressive, and who are strongly supported at home, do well in a day hospital. In my opinion the Department of Health's recommendation that there should be two or three day places for demented patients for every 1000 old people and less than one place for functional illness underestimates the scale of the latter.

Treatments include the administration of drugs and ECT and group therapy, as well as the appropriate regime for such concomitant physical disorders as stroke, arthritis, diabetes and varicose ulcer, though if these dominate the clinical picture a more appropriate place may be a geriatric day hospital. The programme, which should start at 8–9 a.m. and end at 5–6 p.m. consists mainly of occupational therapy—individual and group activities of a recreational or industrial nature. In my experience group activities are the most successful, even though the clientele are far from naturally sociable. Work for others, such as packing for the hospital's sterilisation depot, or collecting and sorting silver paper to raise money for guide dogs for the blind, and sing-songs seem to be especially popular. However, plenty will just want to sit and talk, or sit and sleep. According to the clientele, group therapy, bereavement groups and reality orientation therapy may be included in the programme. Lunch and tea are provided, and as the day hospital is part of the hospital service patients are not allowed to pay for these meals; in my opinion this is a pity, for some old people may feel belittled by not making a contribution to paying their way. All should be encouraged to participate in minor chores such as washing up, and it is particularly beneficial to dependent but fit patients to do things to help others more frail than themselves.

The day hospital is in the charge of a sister or charge nurse who has to be very much aware of the patients and their circumstances and ready to liaise with families and the other community services with which patients are also involved. Often he or she will be the only person who really knows all the clientele, for the doctors spend far less time in the day hospital and may find it impossible to keep fully in touch with as many as 100 patients attending in the course of a week.

Transport is vital for those most in need. Ideally a driver is seconded to the day hospital by the ambulance service, and thus becomes a member of the team and gets to know those whom he collects and their homes very well. He is accompanied by a nurse who helps patients from their homes to the ambulance and supervises them in transit. If she fails to obtain admission she reports back to the sister or charge nurse who then investigates in person or refers the problem to the most appropriate person—relative, social worker, community nurse or GP. Old people who are slow and live upstairs take quite a while to get to the ambulance, and in areas where traffic is dense, or where there is a very extensive territory to be covered, the 'round-up' can take as long as two hours. (Tom Arie has suggested the alternative label of 'transport therapy'). Patients may then only reach the day hospital just in time for lunch, and have to depart straight after 3 o'clock tea.

Bathing and laundering facilities are provided in most day hospitals. By far the most convenient bath is the Medic variety, in which the patient can sit in safety and comfort, without having to be hauled out.

Perhaps under a half of the patients are likely to be discharged to continue life in their own homes without day support. They are acutely ill patients who make a good, swift recovery. Others, however, suffer chronic or frequently relapsing illness, or from very dependent personalities. Some 'discharges,' therefore, are to situations of greater dependency, such as hospital, or a Home though many others are weaned to day centres and thus give place to those in greater need. It is wise if possible to help separate those patients who may be expected to recover, e.g. acutely depressed, from those who probably will not, e.g. the demented. The drug 'Day Hospital' is powerfully addictive!

The patients at a psychogeriatric day hospital, then, have all suffered at least one episode of serious psychiatric illness in late life, and though often lonely this is never the sole reason for their attendance. Some are acutely ill, but for some reason—their own reluctance, the lack of an immediately available bed, or where it seems especially desirable to keep them at home—they are treated as day rather than in-patients. The ability of a day hospital to cope with such problems, provided there are no more than two or three at a time, is remarkable; here day treatment is undoubtedly providing an alternative to admission. Then there are many former inpatients, discharged to the day hospital sooner than would otherwise have been possible and with less likelihood of relapse because of the support they receive there. Depressive patients can be given ECT. Paraphrenics can receive their Stelazine, Modecate or Depixol under supervision. The neurotic and personality disordered are tolerated in a way which is unusual for them outside a psychiatric setting. Demented patients are maintained so that their key supporter can have a regular break, or even go out to work.

Very different models of psychogeriatric day hospitals are those at Mapperly Hospital in Nottingham; Severalls Hospital, in Colchester; and The London Hospital (St Clement's) in Bow. Mapperly in the past took day care perhaps as far as it could go, with a fleet of some 20 ambulances carrying about 400 patients, many of them elderly, to and from the hospital in the course of a seven-day week. Intensive day care together with a very well developed boarding-out scheme reduced the number of hospital beds by as many as there were day places.

In his book *In the service of old age* Anthony Whitehead (1971) describes how Severalls Hospital serves an extensive area of North-East Essex with a day hospital taking 120 psychogeriatric patients a day from within a radius of 20 miles. This, as part of a well organised psychogeriatric service, which also makes special use of intermittent admissions of demented patients, has again allowed a reduction in the number of beds.

The St Clement's Day Hospitals, one established in 1961, the other in 1975, are most usefully situated in the heart of the densely populated London borough which they serve—Tower Hamlets. Each has 30–35 places accommodating as many as 80 patients in the course of a five-day week, none of whom lives more than five miles away. The Day Hospitals, one for high dependency (i.e. mainly demented) patients, providing continuing care and situated within the grounds of St Clement's Hospital, the other for lower dependency (i.e. largely functional patients) most of whom are discharged within two or three months, and located outside the parent hospital in a former chest clinic, are a vital part of a compact but comprehensive psychogeriatric service provided by the London Hospital, also including psychogeriatric assessment beds, a ward for functional patients, another with mainly long-stay patients suffering dementia and, very close at hand, the local authority's special home for the elderly mentally infirm.

Day centres for psychogeriatric patients are provided by some local authorities, sometimes as part of a residential home. They offer supervision and cater for social needs, but provide no medical treatment. Lunch and tea are supplied, at the nominal price charged for Meals on Wheels. Almost all those who attend are brought by a special bus. The clientele is mainly dependent, physically infirm and mildly confused. The main activity is occupational therapy, and much depends on the availability of an occupational therapist, and on her interest and resourcefulness. Baker & Byrne (1977) described the large number of day centres in the community care of psychogeriatric patients in a rural area, Gloucestershire.

Day clubs rarely cater for psychogeriatric patients specifically, but are a social amenity for the elderly, tending to attract the more extraverted. Indeed, the hearty, 'down at the old Bull and Bush' atmosphere of many day clubs is in marked contrast to the silence and somnolence of the average psychogeriatric day hospital.

Luncheon clubs exist mainly to provide meals for those unable or disinclined to cook for themselves, but too fit to require Meals on Wheels; however, they also inevitably encourage a measure of social activity, and appeal to a wider range of personalities than do day clubs.

Sheltered workshops for the elderly are eagerly made use of for the occupation, companionship and small additional income they provide, wherever they have been opened; it seems that as yet there are nowhere near enough to meet the need—something like 100 in the UK, and those mainly in the south-east. Suitable premises are essential, and the manager needs to be able to attract simple factory work and to see that it is performed properly for the unit to be an economic success, and to be able to deal effectively with old people who may be slow and rigid, though generally enthusiastic. Few workshops cater especially for psychogeriatric patients, but they are probably of value in preventing and limiting the depression associated with loss of activity and purpose.

REHABILITATION

Rehabilitation means, literally, restoring ability. One of the first steps in the rehabilitation of the psychogeriatric patient in hospital is to replace dressing-gown and slippers by clothing, preferably his or her own. To be clothed is to be a person once more, not merely a patient, and to wear one's own clothes is a means of asserting one's identity.

In the course of rehabilitation the patient is encouraged to do more and more for himself, even if this means that he goes at a much slower pace than when everything is done for him. Nurses who help patients out of chairs when they are just about able to get up themselves, or wheel the infirm to the dining-table rather than let them spend quarter of an hour getting there, are blocking rehabilitation out of misguided motives of kindness or efficiency. Wards should be so equipped that patients can do as much as possible for themselves. For example most beds should be of divan height, so that the patients (who tend to be small) can get in and out unaided and make their own bed in the morning. The High-Low beds which lower to divan height but can be raised to the level of the traditional hospital bed when the patient requires nursing are especially useful. The ward should be so designed that patients can find their way about, to the lavatories (which should be very clearly marked), the dormitories, their lockers, the dining and day-rooms and the door to the outside. Daily newspapers and topical magazines as well as the inevitable television encourage interest in current affairs. The day and date should be indicated in bold letters and a prominent position, and kept scrupulously accurate. On wards where there are demented patients the staff should continually impart and reiterate basic information about orientation. Open visiting has many advantages, not least that of keeping patients while in hospital in the closest possible contact with their family and friends. Leave for short spells at home, usually at weekends for those with families, mid-week for those who live alone (as community services are minimal at the weekends) is introduced as soon as is practicable. It is important that patients keep some personal possessions, notably false teeth, spectacles and hearing aids. This is far more easily said than done, for if used they are liable to be mislaid, but an efficient marking system helps.

Having some money to spend is almost as important as wearing clothes. So often when patients are first admitted they are penniless, and feel extra helpless; they brought no money in, and their pension book is at once sent away, so for a fortnight or so they may be quite without funds. Every effort should be made to find cash to tide over this difficult period, and later to see that patients get the allowances to which they are entitled. Of course, some grossly confused patients are quite incapable of handling money and lose it as soon as they receive it, but too often those who are able to use it get little or none. A shopping expedition to buy clothing or comforts allows some individuality of choice and helps to restore confidence.

A kitchen and flatlet on the ward or in the occupational therapy department can be used to try out how effectively patients can care for themselves. Subsequently the occupational therapist may take the patient to his or her home, and see how he or she copes there, in the natural environment, as a preliminary to discharge.

Outings to places of interest, especially favourite old haunts in the neighbourhood of the patients' homes, break down the barrier between ward and the community outside and often stimulate lively discussions. And at the very least patients should be taken for a walk away from the ward daily, to sustain interest and mobility. This is especially important for longstay patients, who should not be overlooked in the rehabilitation programme; for them the object is to provide as full a life as is possible in their circumstances, and to slow down the rate of deterioration.

Social activities, such as sing-songs (old songs being particularly evocative of old memories), dances, tea-parties and Bingo sessions may be very heavy going for the staff, but are well worthwhile for the liveliness and lifting of morale they may achieve. It is best if these take place in other places than the patient's own ward sometimes, especially if the ward is for a single sex. It is nice for the men to visit the women, and vice versa, and for both to go to the social centre (if there is one) or occupational therapy department on occasion.

'Keep fit' activities, in addition to individual physiotherapy, can be fun and promote physical activity: ball-throwing round a circle, skittles and even walking-stick hockey are particularly popular.

Rehabilitation may not, of course, always achieve the restoration of ability lost through the diseases of old age, but at least aims to help the patient make the very best use of those abilities which remain.

REFERENCES

Baker A A, Byrne R F J 1977 Another style of psychogeriatric service. Brit J Psychiat 130: 123
Plank D 1979 An overview of the position of elderly people in society. Mind, London
Seebohm Committee 1968 Report of the committee on local authority and allied personal social services, Command 3703. HMSO, London
Whitehead A 1971 In the service of old age. Penguin, Harmondsworth

17

Compulsory treatment

Most elderly patients agree to come into hospital when in need of care and treatment, or at least raise no objection when admission becomes necessary. A minority, however, refuse. They are, of course, quite entitled to do so unless there is good reason to believe that the refusal is the consequence of psychiatric disorder and constitues a serious danger to the patient's health or life, or (rarely) to the safety of others.

Under these circumstances compulsory admission is warranted. In England and Wales the *Mental Health Act* of 1959 applies.

Section 25. This is for observation, over a period of 28 days. Application is made by the next of kin, or more often by a social worker in the employ of the local authority's department of social services, and this is supported by two medical recommendations— one by a doctor having personal knowledge of the patient, usually the general practitioner (though any doctor acting in good faith will do at a pinch), and the other by a doctor with approved experience in psychiatry. These two doctors must not be in partnership with each other, nor on the staff of the same hospital. The two doctors must see the patient within 7 days of each other, and they and the applicant must have done so within 14 days of the day of admission. The certificate is not finally valid until the patient has been officially accepted by the hospital to which he or she is sent, and an officer of the hospital must sign to this effect. During the ensuing 28 days the only person who can discharge the patient is the 'responsible medical officer', which means the consultant psychiatrist into whose bed the admission was made.

Section 29. This is the section most open to abuse, for only one doctor need make the recommendation, and he is not required to have prior knowledge of the patient, though the act indicates that this is desirable. Application and acceptance are as under Section 25. This section, which is for use in an emergency, for it is not always possible to obtain the opinions of two doctors (especially that of a psychiatrist) in a crisis situation, secures admission for 72 hours only.

Three other sections, rarely used, are:

Section 26. This permits compulsory treatment for up to one year. The application and medical recommendations are made as under Section 25, but the two doctors must state their reasons for making the order in some detail, to substantiate the diagnosis of mental illness and explain why informal treatment is not appropriate. After six months the patient has the right to appeal to the Mental Health Review Tribunal (consisting of a lawyer, a doctor and an administrator or social worker, none of whom are on the staff of the hospital) for his release, and in actual practice it is by no means unusual for discharges to be obtained this way.

In none of the foregoing, incidentally, is a magistrate involved. In Scotland, however, the approval of a sheriff is required before any such orders become effective.

Section 60. This is an order made by a magistrate (or judge) and supported by two medical recommendations (as under Section 25) for the compulsory treatment of a patient convicted of a criminal offence.

Section 136. This allows a police officer who finds a person he deems to be mentally disordered in a public place to remove him to a 'place of safety' which is usually (though not necessarily) a psychiatric ward or hospital. This order, like Section 29, is effective for three days.

Compulsory admission accounts for perhaps 5 per cent of those who come into psychogeriatric wards. The remainder are 'informal' patients, with exactly the same rights as patients admitted to any kind of ward, for physical illness. Those most liable to compulsory admission are the paranoid, hypomanic and so severely depressed that they see no justification for treatment. Confused patients, on the other hand, are usually unable sufficiently to comprehend the situation of being admitted to oppose it, and hence are nearly always admitted informally.

The *Mental Health Act* does not permit the compulsory admission of eccentric and personality disordered old people who are not mentally ill or severely subnormal. However, Section 47 of the *Public Health Act* entitles the medical officer of health to make application to his local authority for the compulsory removal to hospital or residential home of anyone who is in a state of serious self-neglect or living in conditions so bad that they endanger health— and some eccentrics and those showing the 'senile squalor syndrome' (p. 00) are dealt with thus. A magistrate must support the removal, and normally the person concerned should be given a week's notice of the action intended; the order then lasts only three weeks.

Disquiet has been expressed about the use of Section 47, e.g. by Gray (1979) and Norman (1980). Well intentioned though the section undoubtedly is, it may be seen as patronising, ageist and an infringement of an older person's right to live as he or she pleases. If squalor and self neglect arise from mental illness, then the *Mental Health Act* may apply; if not, why should not an old person live in privation and filth, as some younger people do, and take an adults responsibility for the consequences, in the form of discomfort or prosecution for creating a nuisance or failure to comply with the terms of a tenancy?

In practice, anyway, Section 47 is very rarely used-on perhaps 300 occasions in the whole of England and Wales in one year.

REFERENCES

Gray F M 1979 Forcing old people to leave their homes. Community Care
  Mental Health Act 1959 HMSO, London
Norman A 1980 Rights and risks. National corporation for the care of old people,
  London

18

The psychogeriatric patient

THE PATIENT'S FAMILY

Far and away the most important agency supporting the psychogeriatric patient at home is the family. There is very little justification for the frequent suggestion that families do less for their old folk than they did. Of course, society has changed considerably in the last 30 years. More women go out to work (the number of the middle aged doing so has increased five fold in the last 50 years), more families live at a distance from each other, and there are more old people. However, for the most part they support their older and more infirm members very well. If they did not, and if the burden of the care of the dependent elderly were to fall on the state, and the health and welfare services, then the hospitals and homes would be so deluged that they would be submerged.

It is, therefore, a vital task of these services (and particularly the social services) to help families carry on giving support. Some practical measures have already been suggested in Chapter 6. Here I shall consider in a little more detail those troubled feelings which families experience towards a psychogeriatric patient which make their work difficult.

Distress over a parent or grandparent who has become add, muddled, irrational or inconsolable is natural and normal, and indeed a necessary part of adjustment to the sickness of a family member. *Bewilderment*, however, when a previously loved mother becomes capricious, suspicious or downright hostile, or a formerly alert and active father is sunk in the depths of gloom, increases distress in a way which is harmful. I remember the shock I felt as a boy when an elderly relative, a pillar of her church, suddenly lost her temper and threw (very inaccurately) a knife at me; I believed that she had turned wicked, and I withdrew from further contact until her funeral a few months later. It was some years afterwards that I appreciated that she had had a stroke and was subject to episodes of confused irritability due to cerebral infarcts. An explanation of the nature of the disorder, and how it affects thinking, mood and behaviour, can give great relief. The course of the malady should also be discussed—whether and how treatment can help, and if not, the rate and pattern of deterioration, and what further measures should be taken at what stages. In the face of depression and paranoia it is important to explain the limitations of argument and exhortation.

Overanxiety on the family's part can blight their own lives and aggravate the patient's condition. For instance, an excessively dutiful daughter may feel that she must be with her mildly demented mother night and day, in case she should fall down, or wander off, or suffer other mishaps for which the daughter could 'never forgive' herself. Consequently she becomes a prisoner to her sense of duty, while the mother feels irked by such unceasing supervision and responds in a peevish manner which heightens the mutual distress. In such cases the daughter needs encouragement and support in doing less for her mother, and in developing a sense of proportion about the degree of disability, in order to conserve her energies for the later stages.

Anger may be a direct reaction to the old person's paranoia, forgetfulness, incontinence or obstinacy; a fury with fate at being so burdened; or keen resentment of other members of the family, or the doctors and social services for not pulling their weight. Overwhelming anger rapidly leads to outright rejection. More often, however, it is suppressed and then contributes to guilt. *Guilt* partly arises from this incompletely acknowledged hostility, and partly from inability to relieve the sick relative's distress or confusion. Prompt practical help may allay anger, while sympathetic discussion can elicit the resentment underlying guilt and the feelings of frustrated 'omnipotence' which give the sense of unworthy failure. When brought out into the open these feelings can be seen in perspective and loom less largely, allowing the realities of the situation to be more clearly grasped.

Sometimes an old person is made a *scapegoat* for family tensions. 'My marriage will break up if Nan doesn't go away', so Nan goes into a home, and three months later the husband runs off with the girl he had been seeing surreptitiously all along. A little girl is so frightened by her confused grandmother who sleeps in the next bedroom that for her sake a place is found for the old lady elsewhere; but the child remains disturbed, and at the child guidance clinic it appears that far more relevant than any fears she had of Grannie are the unspoken hostilities between her parents. Depression or other not immediately diagnosable illness in the key supporting relative may present with the complaint that the old person's vagaries have become insupportable; but what is needed is not removal of the older patient, but treatment for the younger. Domiciliary appraisal and keen social diagnosis are the best techniques for recognising scapegoating and acting to meet the real needs of the situation.

All sorts of workers, notably the social worker, health visitor, general practitioner, community psychogeriatric nurse and informed voluntary workers can help the supporter to sort out these troublesome and disturbing feelings and to manage them. The mutual support provided by relatives' groups (e.g. Fuller et al, 1979) often held in the local day hospital can also be of great value. Noone really knows what it is like to live with a demented old person as well as someone who is actually now doing so, and in an active group feelings can be ventilated and techniques for coping exchanged.

If eventually, however, the old person does go into care, in a hospital or a home, the family still needs help, to make the experience a good rather than a bad one. Grief, guilt, a sense of failure, anxiety and quickness to blame are all common reactions to the admission of an elderly relative who has been looked after with difficulty and strain over a lengthy period at home. The unhappiest outcome is total rejection, which leaves the patient quite bereft and the family deeply scarred. The staff can avert this by showing concern and understanding for the family's feelings, and a readiness to involve them as much as they may wish in continuing care. Open visiting enables close contact to be maintained, and an incidental benefit to the staff is the help which some relatives gladly give to their own and other patients. Again relatives' meetings, for small or larger groups, conducted by the doctor or social worker, or attended by all available staff, may encourage a sharing of feelings which can relieve tension and stimulate mutual support. In such a situation, staff and family are unlikely to find fault with each other for long, but work instead more effectively together for the patients' good.

A group for the relatives of demented patients in the London Hospital (St Clement's) progressed from fury with the nursing and the hospital administration in the first meetings to, on the one hand, concerted action to improve the patients' lot, and, on the other, a thoughtful looking inwards at the troubled feelings aroused by their admission.

Television, radio, newspapers and magazines are now giving some proper attention to the large numbers of the elderly in our society and the problems which may arise from their care. Many programmes and articles are informed and illuminating, but they tend to breadth rather than depth, and are not, of course, always available when the harrassed supporting relative feels urgently in need of comfort and counselling. Excellent approximations to a 'Dr Spock' for the daughter at her wit's end with her deranged and unpredictable mother are Deeping's *Caring for elderly patients* (1979) and the manual by Gray & McKenzie (1980).

THE PSYCHOGERIATRIC PATIENT IN HOSPITAL

The general hospital
In the general hospital, especially the more acute wards which expect a high turnover of patients, the psychogeriatric patient is at risk from *resentment* and *rejection*. The attitude that patients should justify their presence in such a ward by having severe physical illness which will respond to the staff's therapeutic skills is very prevalent, and old people who are simply failing to thrive, and who give an impression of advanced senility are unwelcome. If in addition they are confused or disturbed they may be regarded as a positive danger, and be banished to a side-ward, heavily sedated, to await 'disposal' by a psychiatrist. Often when the psychiatrist visits he finds that virtually none of the information he requires—the duration of the confusion, say, the mode of onset, the actual reason for admission, the social circumstances—has been obtained. He may see in bold writing the diagnosis 'senile dementia' written as a final judgement.

Quite often old people are admitted to medical or surgical wards as emergencies which turn out to be social rather than medical. This arouses considerable ire, and referrals of the elderly tend to be regarded with dark suspicion. Yet more than half of those in the average general medical or orthopaedic ward most of the time are 65 or considerably more. Old age is, after all, the period of highest morbidity, when people who have never been seriously ill in their lives before have to come into hospital. The elderly need all the resources of the modern general hospital as much as, if not more than, anybody else, but they are often allowed them very grudgingly.

Those who are physically ill and mentally alert tend to get good treatment, but if they are depressed or peculiar or confused (but quiet) or if progress is slow or absent after the first fortnight, a pattern of neglect and rejection sets in. They are referred for 'disposal' to the geriatrician, psychiatrist or old people's homes, and while waiting what is felt to be an unconscionably long time, receive only basic physical care from the nurses, little or no rehabilitation and no attention from the doctor beyond the occasional grumble: 'Is she still here?' Sometimes indignation explodes in a totally unrealistic discharge home, at the insistence of a consultant with no knowledge of the conditions there, refusing to use his imagination to visualise just how this patient could possibly manage anywhere alone, and the bewildered old person is sent off at half a day's notice into an unprepared and dismayed community, only to 'bounce' into the lap of the geriatrician or psychiatrist a day or two later—that is, if she survives. (It sometimes seems to me that an important role of the geriatrician is to protect surgeons and other physicians from awareness of their failures.)

Psychogeriatric problems are so prevalent that they cannot be left to the psychiatrists and geriatricians. All doctors and nurses who have to do with old people (and that means all clinicians except perhaps paediatricians and obstetricians) need to have some knowledge of psychogeriatrics and a readiness to deal with the human problems inextricably mixed with the medical problems which come their way. The example they set their staff in this respect is likely to be taken up, with a consequent improvement in attitudes and the quality of care. Doctors' attitudes, though, are largely shaped by their training, and until geriatrics and psychogeriatrics are given their proper place in the curricula of the medical schools and teaching hospitals too many doctors will neither know nor wish to know about the aged a people as well as patients.

The geriatric hospital

A high proportion of the patients in a geriatric ward have significant psychiatric disorder as well as, or even rather than, physical infirmity. Dementia is especially common, usually but not invariably associated with difficulty in walking, to warrant the placement in a geriatric rather than a psychiatric ward. Depression (of moderate severity, manifest as apathy more often than anxiety) and personality disorder are also prominent, as well as paranoia arising in various ways.

The accommodation in geriatric hospitals is sometimes the worst possible. Buildings tend to be former workhouses, with a grim exterior which no amount of improvement to the inside can really offset. For the elderly patients they still have the workhouse image. Fortunately there have been substantial improvements in Britain in the last five years with some new as well as up-graded wards.

The turnover of patients is relatively low, for many are chronic and stay for a year or more. In the hospital service, low turnover is equated with low status, and a difficulty in attracting staff or getting an adequate share of finance and amenities. Consequently there are generally too few people to do the work, which many find unrewarding. By no means all the staff are well suited to what they are supposed to do. Morale, therefore, is precarious and, under the pressure of addition to the work load, changes in policy and senior staff, and heavy criticism, can readily slip.

The patients are very much the serious casualties of late life. Their disabilities are either so great that they cannot be cared for outside hospital, or they are so old, or have been so solitary or difficult, that when they become infirm there is none outside an institution to look after them. However at any one time there will be quite a large number of frail but not seriously infirm old people quite fit to reside in an old people's home if a place ever becomes available to them. Unfortunately, such places go first to those in need in the community, and those already accommodated in hospital, even unsuitably, especially in the less acute beds, are given a lowish priority.

Particularly in a geriatric hospital patients are likely to be institutionalised. Institutionalisation has been called by Dr Russell Barton 'a mental bedsore'. The features include apathy, lack of individuality and undue submissiveness. Regimentation, overmedication, lack of personal choice and belongings, lack of social stimulation and a purpose in life, and prolonged inactivity contribute to the disorder.

While it is good geriatric practice to keep patients as mobile as possible, geriatric wards are not really designed for those who wander about restlessly. Such patients tend to be transformed into more suitable candidates for the place they are in after a few weeks, or months, by being heavily sedated and locked into geriatric chairs.

I do not agree with those of my psychiatrist colleagues who claim that the care of the severely demented, whose disability is due to organic brain disease and is irreversible, should be in geriatric rather than psychiatric wards. On the whole psychiatric wards are better designed for the task (they usually have quite a lot of legroom) and psychiatric staff better trained to deal with difficult aggressive confused wanderers without recourse to excessive restraint. Besides geriatric hospitals already have more than enough to cope with in the physically infirm. However, there is a great deal to be said for the staff of each kind of hospital's getting some experience in the others field. This may be by secondment during training, and also by regular visits for consultation by the psychiatrist to the geriatric wards, and the geriatrician to the psychiatric hospital.

The psychiatric hospital

In 1949, 11 per cent of the general population were over 65 years of age, and 27 per cent of those in psychiatric hospitals; in 1960, the proportions were 12 per cent and 37 per cent respectively. The trend has continued, so that in most psychiatric hospitals today more than half the female patients and one third of the male are over 65. Many of these are chronic schiozphrenics, who were admitted years ago in their youth, before the days of active, effective treatment and rehabilitation. They are thoroughly institutionalised, their former homes no longer exist, in many cases, and they have lost contact with their families and the community in which they used to live. They are a hardy, eccentric group who need very little care until they become physically infirm with ageing. They have become well adjusted to life in a mental hospital, and are often useful in carrying out ward chores. Their numbers are slowly dwindling as they die and are not replaced, for schizophrenia is now treated in acute and rehabilitation wards, and supposedly managed thereafter in the community. It is not policy to attempt to move such patients, for whom the hospital has become their home, elsewhere; but a few are satisfactorily discharged to group homes, five or six carefully selected patients being accommodated together in a house and supervised by a visiting doctor, nurse and social worker.

A larger number, now, of those over 65 are suffering from severe dementia, and it is this group, increasing all the time, which taxes the hospital most. Far less able to care for themselves than any other class of patients, they tax nursing resources while offering no prospect of their discharge or even improvement (Early & Nicholas, 1981).

In this situation there sometimes develops a split between the acute admission wards for younger patients and the wards for the demented. The former have plenty of action and a high turnover, with a relatively high ratio of staff to patients, and are where most of the doctors spend most of their time. The wards for the demented, on the other hand, are truly 'back' wards, away from the centre of things, even lacking such basic facilities as proper ablutions and heated lavatories, where a small group of nurses struggles grimly with an oppressive load of incontinent, helpless, lost old people, visited by a reluctant junior doctor perhaps once a week, and by the consultant and other staff hardly ever. Small wonder,

then, that depression, defeatism and bitterness are prevalent among
the staff (let alone the patients) of the wards for the demented.
They feel cut off from the mainstream of psychiatry, which was
what most of them wished to do; and they lack even the facilities of
a geriatric hospital—physiotherapy, and doctors who are really up
to date in their knowledge of medicne—when their charges become
physically disabled and ill.

As has been explained in Chapter 12, the development of a
psychogeriatic firm within the hospital does much to lessen these
ills, by organising a group with a special concern for the elderly. A
visiting geriatrician, or better still, one who has some beds of his
own within the psychiatric hospital (Drs Lodge and Parnell have
written of their work in Leicester and Birmingham mental hospitals respectively) can help considerably too. But, as has already been
stated, the problems of elderly patients with psychiatric disability
are so prevalent that they cannot be left to the geriatricians, or even
the psychogeriatricians. It is every consultant and senior nursing
officer's duty to support the staff working in all his or her wards,
which means visiting regularly and reliably, seeing the problems
for themselves, meeting the staff, listening to their grievances
(many of which will, however unfairly, be against him for his relative neglect of the ward), helping them to sort out fantasy from
fact, encouraging good work and tactfully improving that which is
bad, promoting understanding of the ward's role in the range of
services provided for the elderly, stimulating interest and crossfer-
tilisation by arranging visits to other units, and using the full
weight of his authority to improve conditions wherever he sees the
chance of doing so.

THE PSYCHOGERIATRIC PATIENT IN THE RESIDENTIAL HOME

Old people's homes in Britain may be private, voluntary or statu-
tory Part Three accommodation provided by the local authorities
for the infirm elderly in their communities. Private homes are
beyond the means of all but a few; if care and supervision are to be
provided, rather than just board and lodgings, the cost will be at
the very least £100 per week (which is, incidentally, considerably
less than that of keeping a patient in a National Health Service
hospital). Even private homes have considerable staffing difficulties. I have known those where none except the matron has more
than the merest smattering of English, and none any training at all.

Voluntary homes, which vary a good deal in quality, usually cater for special groups, such as ex-servicemen, or seamen, or are under the auspices of a religious body such as the Church of England or the Salvation Army (though not necessarily requiring residents to hold any particular faith).

However, the great majority of old people's homes are in Part Three accommodation. This has evolved from the days of the Poor Law, and workhouses for paupers, and it is relatively recently that the workhouse image has been thrown off. Time was when many homes were Dickensian institutions, with little regard for privacy, personal possessions or self-determination, in which the sexes were segregated so that couples were parted. In the last decade or two, however, there has been a transformation, so that most homes are now purpose-built (often most imaginatively) or former country houses, providing single rooms for many, individual lockers, wardrobes and washbasins, and rarely requiring residents to sleep more than four to a room. Attitudes have changed, too, so that the rights of the residents are scrupulously safeguarded.

The problems which arise, though, are not due to the buildings but to the people in them. Staff are usually insufficient and untrained (care assistants in London are strikingly less well trained than nursing aides working in homes in New York, according to (Godlove et al, 1980), and the residents are so infirm as to need a fair amount of care. I have sometimes, cynically, reflected that from the point of view of some staff the ideal resident is someone who should not be in a home at all. Old people who are capable of caring for themselves should be in their own homes, supported by families and the community services, or in sheltered housing. The clientele of a residential home are bound to differ from the elderly in the community by being older, more isolated (by age or 'difficult' personality) and more infirm. Matrons who have worked in homes for many years comment that there are far more decrepit, awkward and confused residents than there used to be. This is true, and should be so, but it presents a challenge to the staff. Up to one half of the residents of ordinary residential homes in Britain are significantly handicapped by dementia (Masterton et al, 1979).

It is not expected that homes should provide nursing care, as a rule, but simply as much help as a family would be expected to give an old and feeble or muddled relative. It is reasonable that homes should cope with those who are confused, but not forever wandering away and getting lost, or persistently aggressive, or doubly incontinent, just as they cope with those who can get about with some help, but do not have to be carried everywhere. However, where so many elderly people in need are gathered together, and the staff (who are, after all, neither their friends nor relatives) have no special knowledge of how to cope with them, problems do arise.

A great deal depends on the matron and warden. At one time I found that half the referrals from 50 homes in the area covered by the service which I was associated came from one source: this had very little to do with the clientele, but much with the difficulties the matron was having in tolerating them and managing her staff. One soon gets to know which homes cope best with particular kinds of residents—and this has less to do with the number of staff than their personalities. Cries of 'Half my staff will resign if this old lady isn't removed', or 'All the residents are up in arms about her' are strongly suggestive that the person complained of is a scapegoat for all sorts of tensions within the home, and that if she is simply removed another will soon be found.

Staff usually approach their work with goodwill, and are sometimes dismayed, hurt or aggrieved when it is not returned. A resident may then be condemned as not merely difficult, but 'impossible', and treated as such, which can lead to such a rapid deterioration in the relationship that before long the old person's behaviour *is* impossible for the home, and the case for removal seems incontrovertible. When a resident barricades him or herself in a room and fights off all comers, the reason is far less often that he or she has become acutely psychotic than that this is the ultimate outcome of mishandling and aggravation. Spontaneous emotional reactions to rude, querulous or aggressive old people, and the need to establish that 'you're wrong—because I'm staff and must be right', can make matters very much worse.

Selection of potential staff or 'care assistants' with the maturity, stability, good humour and genuine care for the elderly which the work ideally requires is, of course, desirable, but not always practicable, for in many areas there are too few applicants to permit much picking and choosing. Where there is a shortage of all grades of nurses for geriatric and psychogeriatric wards, it is hardly surprising that there should be still fewer candidates for residential homes, where the work does not even have the status conferred by the title 'nurse'. Modern, purpose-built homes have been opened and then remained half-empty for months because too few people have been found to staff them.

Some form of in-service training, however, should be provided for the matrons, wardens, and their assistants by every local authority. This may take the form of a course of half-days during which formal lectures are given (though unfortunately some care assistants will not co-operate unless they are paid extra afterwards for having had some formal training), there are visits to various units in the geriatric and psychogeriatric services, and there is a great deal of informal free discussion under the guidance of a seasoned matron or social worker. I feel, too, that regular staff meetings within the homes, along the lines of those held in some hospitals wards (Ch. 13. p. 147) could be of value in helping staff to learn from their experience and in dealing with the tensions which so readily arise between themselves and the residents, and each other. The sharing of anger, anxiety, unhappiness and antagonism in such a setting allows these feelings to be discussed and understood rather than simply acted upon. There are powerful fantasies associated with the idea of madness which can be evoked in the inexperienced and untrained by encounters with even the very elderly mentally disturbed; I have never yet met a dangerous psychogeriatric patient, though I am always being told about them. Staff meetings help to correct alarmist fantasies by reminding all of the realities of the situation; for example, though Mr Smith may lash out with his stick when he is crossed, he is 90 years old, has not much strength in his arms, and the very fact that he needs a stick indicates that he is unlikely to pursue anyone very energetically.

Except in the occasional cases of serious psychiatric illness, drugs are not widely useful in the treatment of psychogeriatric disorder in the residential home, which mainly consists of dementia and mild to moderate depression. When I confessed to a group of matrons that when I prescribed a small dose of a tranquilliser sometimes it was not because I thought it would directly benefit the patient but might be of some comfort to the staff, one of them confessed in return that often she and her colleagues did not give the drugs prescribed as they knew they were no good! Such games are a rather poor substitute for acceptance, understanding and a regime which offers residents stimulation and distraction from their anxious bewilderment and unhappy preoccupations. Bustle, activity and comings and goings are rather exceptional in residential homes, where too often the old people sit about, silent or asleep, rousing only for meals, bed or a squabble over 'who's been sitting in my chair?' Occupational therapists are, alas, rare birds these days, but where available they have a most useful part to play in promoting activities within homes. Visiting should be encouraged, without much rigidity over hours, and outings, shopping expeditions and social functions urged. I believe, too, that community meetings attended by all the residents and all available staff could be a valuable forum for discussion and the discharge of discontent (see Ch. 15, p. 166).

Commonly the staff of the residential homes feel isolated, left to their own devices, uninformed and liable to more criticism than credit. They comment that the social worker who was dealing with a difficult old person in the community drops right out of the picture once he or she becomes a resident. While the social services departments are seriously stretched, an elderly client may well assume a lower priority once in care, but the continuation of support to settle him or her in is likely to provide a boost to the morale of the home as well as help to the individual. In this respect the best practice in the United States appears to surpass that in Britain. Also, the senior social workers in charge of the overall administration of the homes have an important duty to keep in close touch, and be seen to care. This does not mean taking every complaint at face value, and being a party to moving on the hapless bunch of misfits who tend to be trundled from one home to another in so many boroughs, but looking at problems in depth and helping homes to contain them. The role is strictly comparable to that of a hospital consultant supporting his long-stay wards.

Visits by a psychogeriatrician are generally sporadic, in response to the GP's request that one of his patients, who happens to be a resident, be seen, but there is usually the opportunity for a discussion with the matron about the difficulties experienced with this particular old person which may lead on to more general matters. Ideally, as there is such a high morbidity in the homes, there should be regular visits for general consultation and for assessment of individual residents who are causing concern, but most psychiatrists and psychogeriatricians have too little time to be able to spare much for this purpose. At the least, though, there might be a regular meeting between the psychogeriatrician and the senior social worker at which areas of special need could be identified and examined.

Most areas now have one or two special homes for the elderly mentally infirm (EMI) which cater mainly for the demented, but usually also include one or two particularly difficult old people. Such homes are relatively well staffed, both in respect of numbers and training (often the matron and warden are psychiatric nurses) and may or may not be specially designed. In Redruth, Cornwall, there is a most interesting EMI home, shaped like a boomerang, with an observation centre in the middle of the upper floor from which all parts of the home can be overseen; it is placed next to a

day centre for subnormal children, and is thus much less of a re-
treat than are many homes. The clientele are exactly the same as
those one meets in the 'demented' wards of any psychiatric hospital
and very few staff have any training, but there are plenty of them
(drawn from an area in which there is little competition from in-
dustry) and they show considerable tolerance and goodwill. So
much better does the resident's lot seem to be, indeed, than if
accommodated in hospital, that one is prompted to ask whether, if
there were more such homes, any demented old people would really require hospital care.

However, while psychogeriatricians tend to favour EMI homes
(when they can be closely linked to an active psychogeriatric service), sociologists (e.g. Meacher, 1972) and directors of social services tend to frown upon such segration, and point out the risks of
stigmatisation and unduly low expectation of the reisent's capaci-
ties. Alternative suggestions are an EMI wing or floor within an
ordinary old people's home or a complete mix of residents in the
hope that the more able will help the less and will gain self esteem
by so doing. (This may work if the mix is right: if there are large
numbers of the confused those who are not so may wonder, 'Am I
the only sane one her? And for how long?')

The 'hotel' model of residential care has been decried by Lipman
& Slater (1977) who instead advocate an 'apartment' approach where
the residents generally look after themselves but approach the staff
as caretakers (or janitors) rather as managers, so that the staff's role
is not to run the services for the residents but to help out in time of
need. This sounds very like the role of the warden in sheltered
housing and might be less appropriate in a home unless the residents were unusually able.

The nursing home which has flourished since the Medicare programme in the United States has no exact equivalent for the most
part in Britain. It occupies a place intermediate between the residential home and the geriatric or psychogeriatric ward with more
nursing than is usual in the former but less specialised medical
supervision than in the latter. Misgivings about their functioning
were on the whole alleviated by a report of the Joint Information
Service of the America Psychiatric Association and Mental Health
Association, *Old folks at homes* (Glasscote et al, 1976).

Arguments about the amount of health care which should be
available in residential homes and how much the residents should
be left to run their own lives continue and are generally valuable in
preventing the residents from being neglected or overprotected. It
must be recognised, though, that in Britain at any rate, being of

pensionable age is not early enough to secure admission to a Home and the usual ticket is considerable infirmity. Homes do not very often make their residents physically or mentally infirm, but are places to which the infirm tend to go.

REFERENCES

Barton 1966 Institutional neurosis, 2nd edn. Wright, Bristol
Deeping E 1979 Caring for elderly parents. Constable, London
Early D, Nicholas M J 1981 Two decades of change. Glenside Hospital population surveys 1960–80. Brit Med J 1: 1446
Fuller J, Ward E, Evans A, Gardner A, Massam K 1979 Dementia support groups for relatives. Brit Med J 1: 1684
Glasscote R, Beigel A, Butterfield J A, Clare E, Cox B, Elders R, Gudeman J E, Gurel L, Lewis R, Miles D, Raybin J, Reifler C, Vito E 1976 Old folks at homes. Joint information service of the American psychiatric association and mental health association, Washington
Godlove C, Dunn G, Wright H 1980 Caring for old people in London and New York: the 'nurses aids' interview. J Royal Soc Med 73: 713
Gray F M, McKenzie H 1980 Taking care of your elderly relative. Allen & Unwin, London
Lipman A, Slater R 1977 Homes for old people towards a positive environment. The Gerontologist 17: 146
Masterton G, Holloway E M, Timbury G 1979 The prevalence of organic cerebral impairment and behavioural problems within local authority homes for the elderly. Age and Ageing 8: 226
Meacher M 1972 Taken for a ride. Longman, Harlow
Parnell R W 1968 Prospective geriatric bed requirements in a mental hospital. Geront Clin 10: 30

19

Training

Until very recently *doctors* have been taught astonishingly little psychiatry and geriatrics in their undergraduate years. When one considers that a third of the patients attending a doctor's surgery are likely to be doing so because of emotional disorder, that almost half the hospital beds in this country are occupied by psychiatric patients, and that so much of the work of general hospitals is concerned with the aged, the neglect of these specialties by the teaching hospitals has been little less than scandalous. The situation has improved as regards psychiatry lately (though most students still spend less than one-tenth of their clinical training on this vast, complex and desperately important subject) but geriatrics remains very much the poor relation of medicine, and psychogeriatrics (and mental subnormality) are the Cinderellas of psychiatry. At the time of writing there are only two or three chairs of geriatric medicine in London, with its twelve undergraduate medical schools, every one of which has two or more professors of general medicine. In the whole of Britain there is but one professor who is, and practices as, a clinical psychogeriatrician, at Nottingham.

A vicious circle is set up whereby students who are taught little or no geriatrics, and instead pick up the contemptuous attitudes of their teachers, become doctors who despise the subject, avoid it as much as possible, and, where they cannot, practise it badly, thus setting their juniors as bad an example as that which they themselves received, and discouraging recruitment to a field which, however needy, will never attract as many people as are required. The current moves towards improving the hospital and health services for the elderly and the mentally ill and handicapped owe very little to the teaching hospitals, and far more to public consternation over the neglect exposed by the book *Sans Everything*, and hospital enquiries into scandals which could not be ignored up and down the country.

Psychogeriatrics is usually taught in the context of psychiatry, though at Nottingham, where there is an integrated Department of

Health in Old Age, and in Manchester, where geriatrics and psychiatry are taught concurrently, the close relationship to geriatric medicine is made very plain. Most London teaching hospitals have now appointed a consultant psychiatrist with a special interest in the elderly, eager to teach, but often restricted by lack of teaching time and facilities. For example, if the department of psychiatry serves no defined catchment area and tends not to have older patients in the main teaching hospital unit where the medical students are mainly taught, then the psychogeriatrician will either have to wrest them away to a peripheral hospital where there are suitable patients to be seen, or be content with the odd lecture or demonstration which may hardly give enough emphasis to the importance the subject will take on for them after they qualify.

The London Hospital, however, takes full responsibility for the population of the borough in which it is situated, and consequently medical students have the opportunity of learning something about psychogeriatrics in an area with which they are familiar. Seminars, visits to the psychogeriatric assessment unit, day hospital and wards for functional and for confused patients (some of whom are long-stay as there is no provision for such patients elsewhere) and, above all, domiciliary visiting with the consultant, give them an inkling of the subject.

Psychiatrists in training are fortunate if they learn anything worthwhile about the psychiatry of old age without serving on a psychogeriatric firm. In hospitals where there is such a firm, then the only experience in the field is to be obtained on it. In those, without, the likelihood that the general psychiatrist will have an interest in the special problems and management of his older patients which he will communicate to his juniors is unfortunately slender (though in fact I developed my interest this way). Ideally, no psychiatrist should reach consultant status (or be eligible to sit the examination for Membership of the Royal College of Psychiatrists) without having served six months on a psychogeriatric firm. The Royal College of Psychiatrists in Britain has lately stipulated that senior registrar posts must include a substantial experience in the psychiatry of old age to be recognised for training.

On the psychogeriatric firm the trainee learns about the physical, psychological and social aspects of ageing, and how these affect psychiatric morbidity. There is an opportunity to observe the interaction of hereditary, organic and environmental influence, and the multiplicity of diagnoses in old age, while learning to sort the relevant from the coincidental. Visits to patient's homes open up new insight in those whose experience of psychiatry has been confined to hospital, and the discovery may be made that in psychogeriatrics work with the patient's family can especially be stimulating and rewarding. It may also be a surprise to find that the principles of psychotherapy can be applied to the elderly, and that vigorous treatment of the severe depressive by physical means is neither harsh nor foolhardy, but very necessary. The wide variety of agencies involved with the elderly needs to be understood, and the problems of communication pondered. If the value of team-work has not been appreciated previously, it will be learned now, as the relative helplessness of doctors and nurses without the com-plementary skills of social workers, occupational therapists and physiotherapists becomes apparent.

The Appendix on pages 211–213 is a scheme for taking the history of and examining the psychogeriatric patient which may be helpful to the psychiatrist in training, not least by indicating all possible lines of action once the assessment has been made.

The formation of a Group for the Psychiatry of Old Age within the Royal College of Psychiatrists in 1973 was timely, and its recog-nition as a full Section of the College three years later (even though recognition as a sub-specialty of psychiatry has so far been with-held) has boosted the education of psychiatrists in training, of potential psychogeriatricians and of those who already call them-selves such. There are similar encouraging trends within the Amer-ican and Canadian Psychiatric Associations and the Royal College of Psychiatrists in Australia and New Zealand. This is to the advantage of psychiatry in general, for the psychogeriatrician has as good a claim as any (and as strong a need) to be considered a com-plete psychiatrist.

The *geriatrician* needs to learn some psychiatry if he is not be at a loss with many of his patients. In the past geriatricians have been trained mainly, if not solely, in general medicine, which made them excellent physicians but indifferent psychiatrists; for betwixt general medicine and psychiatry, it often seems, is a great gulf—a gulf due less to any lack of goodwill than to attitude and orienta-tion. The geriatrician with no grounding in psychiatry may not rec-ognise the many faces of depression, and will not be familiar with the concepts of ambivalence, projection and denial which are so common in the reactions of elderly patients to their disabilities and in the relationships they make. Ideally, any consultant geriatrician should have had at least six months' experience on a psychogeriat-ric firm—and every consultant psychogeriatrician six months' in-struction in geriatrics. An exchange of registrar or senior registrars in the respective specialties for the period could be an excellent arrangement.

The other group of doctors in special need of extra instruction in psychogeriatrics are the *general practitioners*, who are far more often consulted about the problems of the elderly than anyone else. Obviously the more they can learn at postgraduate courses (which they are encouraged to attend) the better, and any psychogeriatrician worth his salt will take every opportunity of promoting his subject at lectures, seminars and demonstrations. The domiciliary visit is another useful form of training, when GP and psychiatrist meet and see the patient together at home and consult afterwards; unfortunately, such are the exigencies of modern practice that usually when the specialist is free to call, in the evening, the GP is busy with his surgery. Thirdly, these days quite a few GPs are employed in hospitals as part-time clinical assistants, and those who are thus members of the psychogeriatric team should be in a position to acquire some training as well as experience.

I have given first place in this chapter to the training of doctors because they exert considerable influence, by example, precept and policy-making.

The instruction given *psychiatric nurses* in Britain according to the Registered Mental Nurse's syllabus is admirable, but this can be offset by their actual expereince in demoralised 'back wards'. Unless the teaching on these wards is in keeping with that of the training-schools, the student nurse may become disillusioned, and be lost to the hospital service after qualification. It is important to keep sisters and charge nurses abreast of current trends by frequent study days and vistis to other wards and units; there must be time to discuss what they see and speak from their own experience. Where there is a psychogeriatric firm the nurses working on it should be well informed.

General nurses have, in the past, known far too little about mental health considering the frequency with which they encounter psychiatric problems (e.g. confusional states and psychosomatic disorders, to say nothing of the 10 per cent of patients in general medical wards having taken overdoses) but recently their syllabus (for the SRN and SEN diplomas) has been revised, so that all should receive instruction and experience in psychiatry (and geriatrics). In practice this means that if there are psychogeriatric wards the 'learner' nurses will probably not go to them, as they are seen as too 'geriatric' for the psychiatric training and too 'psychiatric' for the geriatric, so that a nurse may complete her training with no experience of the management of a difficult demented old person, or a dehydrated elderly depressive!

Occupational therapists receive a very good grounding in psychiatry, which shows in the insight and understanding they bring to their work in general and geriatric as well as psychiatric hospitals. The quality of their psychogeriatric experience, however, varies a good deal with the hospitals to which they are seconded during training, and is likely to be more organised and stimulating where there is a psychogeriatric firm. Some therapists working in psychiatric units are especially keen on psychotherapeutic techniques such as group therapy and psychodrama, and on reality orientation and behaviour therapy. Those based on geriatric units are more attuned to overcoming the psychological obstacles to rehabilitation, restoring confidence and teaching techniques for coping with daily living activities.

From an early stage in their careers *physiotherapists* are likely to be faced with the problem of patients who make poor progress in rehabilitation for no very clear physical reason. Until recently, physiotherapists have not had much to do with psychiatric wards or hospitals, but the development of psychogeriatrics is involving them more and more. They have to learn to adapt their techniques to the psychogeriatric patient, whose co-operation cannot be taken for granted however much she may need help. In my experience, most physiotherapists who 'take the plunge' into psychiatry learn fast and contribute a great deal. Happily, more and more are doing so.

Speech therapists have much to offer the elderly, but deal with relatively few. I have been particularly impressed by the benefits of a group approach to stroke victims with speech problems. In future speech and occupational therapists and physiotherapists in Britain will share a basic training with, it is hoped, full recognition of the needs for an opportunities in work with the elderly.

Clinical psychologists are trained in testing mental ability which theoretically is very relevant to work with the elderly, but in practice most psychologists now are not very keen on testing, and find old subjects among the least satisfactory to test. Therapy is much more interesting to many psychologists, and the value of behaviour therapy in the management of psychiatric disorders in late life is only just beginning to be appreciated. Psychologists in training need some special experience in geriatric psychiatry, to learn what they can contribute and how welcome they are to the psychogeriatric team.

Social workers at present consist largely of those with little formal training but much practical experience with the elderly, those with a generic training, applicable to all ages and situations, but as yet little experience, and not a few with neither training nor experience. In Britain, since the reorganisation of the social services, those of the former who used to specialise in the problems of older clientele are, like the previous mental welfare and child care officers, no longer specialists, but may be called upon for any form of social work. The younger, generically trained workers do not specialise either; they are concerned with the elderly only through an emergency involving an old person on a day when they are 'on call', or if they are allocated older clients among their many younger ones. In Chapter 16 I have expressed misgivings about this arrangement, and it is my impression that in some departments the influence of those with any deep knowledge and understanding of the problems of mental health in old age is small. It is earnestly to be hoped that directors will recognise the importance of training their workers to deal with such problems by making full use of the 'nous' of the more seasoned staff, encouraging some of those who are trained to specialise in work with the elderly, encouraging visits to and from hospitals and ensuring that trainees under supervision apply the standards of casework to the elderly as well as the young.

In conclusion, I will mention the *Health Advisory Service*, the Hospital Centre, Mind, Age Concern, and the National Corporation for the Care of Old People, organisations which, in Britain, have contributed substantially to training.

The former is a group of experts commissioned by the Minister of Health to visit all psychiatric and geriatric units in England and Wales. Thus they are in a unique position to compare standards and to promote good practice. They are not, as some had feared, a hostile inspectorate, but a truly advisory body whose criticisms are usually informed and instructive, and whose visits only do psychogeriatrics and its teaching good.

The *Hospital Centre* is an invaluable establishment, set up by the admirable King's Fund to inform and stimulate the hospitals and those who use them. It has done excellent work in arranging study days, discussions, publications and exhibitions on psychogeriatrics, rightly recognising that this is one of the most important yet neglected of the hospital services. Truly, at times one feels that the Centre shines like a good deed in a naughty world.

The work of *Mind* and *Age Concern* has been mentioned in Chapter 3. To the establishment Mind sometimes seems a maverick organisation which makes too many waves, but they are definitely on the side of the patient, and as far as the elderly are concerned their hearts are securely in the right place. They, together with

Age Concern and the *National Corporation for the Care of Old People*, have produced many useful publications mainly for a lay readership, have sponsored some research into patterns and problems of care and have organised several multi disciplinary conferences and more specialised courses, e.g. for the staffs of residential homes.

Addresses

Age Concern: Bernard Sunley House, 60 Pitcairn Road, Mitcham, Surrey CR4 3LL.

British Geriatrics Society: Bernard Sunley House, 60 Pitcairn Road, Mitcham, Surrey CR4 3LL.

Health Advisory Service: Sutherland House, Sutton, Surrey.

Hospital Centre: (King's Fund Centre): 126 Albert Street, London NW1.

National Corporation for the Care of Old People: Nuffield Lodge, Regents Park, London NW1 4RS

Royal College of Psychiatrists (Section for the Psychiatry of Old Age): 17 Belgrave Square, London SW1.

20

Conclusion

Psychiatry was caught unawares by the number and needs of the elderly mentally ill, which have become so pressing in the past 30 years. Gradually, however, special psychiatric services are being developed for the elderly, and a new subspecialty, psychogeriatrics, is gaining recognition wherever the elderly population exceeds seven per cent or so.

Pressure has come not only from within the mental hospitals, but from general and geriatric wards perplexed by confusion, depression and disturbed behaviour in their older patients, from social services departments coping with more old people than they feel they have the means or knowledge to handle, and from the community at large, ultimately finding a voice for its concern in the Minister or Secretary of State for Health. In Britain and elsewhere priorities and allocations have been revised, to try to ensure that the elderly and the mentally ill and handicapped get their fair share of finance and facilities. At the same time, the autonomy of local health authorities and the drastic shortage of funds where the economy is depressed and the Health Service funding is anyway chronically inadequate means that guidance from the centre or on high is not always heeded. An articulate and effective body representing the consumer (like the Community Health Councils in Britain only with more teeth) is thus needed to express public concern and see that the limited resources are properly distributed.

But how are these resources best to be used? What is good psychogeriatric practice? The principles described in Chapters 12 and 13 are broadly correct, but different services vary quite a lot while claiming to be effective. Are they deceiving themselves? Or do places, populations, patterns of existing provision and personalities make all the difference? It is pretty obvious that arrangements where people are widely dispersed in a rural district must be modified from those which suit an inner city borough, while the new buildings and new population in a new town present different opportunities and new challenges. The Goodmayes service originally described by Arie (1971) had no day hospital, nor has that in the Southampton area as explained by Godber (1978). Yet Baker & Byrne (1977) are such keen advocates of day treatment and care that they claimed that the numbers of beds recommended by the Department of Health and Social Security might be excessive. I (Pitt & Silver, 1980) am very committed to the close integration with the geriatric service achieved by working together in a joint unit but most of my colleagues seem to manage just as well without such an arrangement.

A most important question is: how much can be achieved by community care, and how much requires some kind of institution? Supplementary questions are: who should be giving the community care (e.g. the primary health care team led by the general practitioner, the community physician and his staff, the social workers and social services, out reach from psychiatric and geriatric hospitals, or neighbourly or organised volunteers)? And what kind of institutions—acute, community, mental or geriatric hospitals, residential or nursing homes?

There is a great need for operational research (Arie & Isaacs, 1978) which will clearly and carefully evaluate the problems to be solved, the effects of culture and tradition, population structure, affluence, transport, the quality and quantity of hospital accommodation and homes, the attitudes of administrators and other professionals, and the resources of staff, space and beds made available to the psychogeriatric service, and then assess how well these problems are solved. How quickly are problems referred, and how promptly assessed, and how appropriate is the action then determined and what delay is there before before it is taken and how effective are the results in terms of improving the patient's condition and situation, and for how long? What needs are not met by the service and who else perforce meets them (e.g. the geriatrician, the orthopaedic surgeon with his beds 'blocked' by demented old ladies who have taken a tumble, residential homes taking sick old people in a crisis)? What needs are not met at all and what is the consequence for the sufferers and the strain on their families? This form of research is laborious and fairly costly but should pay for itself if it gets the right answers to the right questions.

Dementia research is also vital, and is fortunately proceeding apace in many centres, with added urgency as the tidal wave of the very old threatens existing services, and dementia threatens so dreadfully the last years of the many of us who may now expect to be old. Whether an answer will be found, when, and in what form (e.g. a biochemical remedy or a prophylactic life style) remain very uncertain, but the sense of isolation so many pioneers in geriatric psychiatry and geriatrics felt when facing the problems of dementia a few years ago has been relieved; almost everybody, it seems, wants to know about dementia now!

It is still frustrating, though, to work in a specialist field which is not fully recognised. I had a visitor recently from a Far Eastern capital who wanted to set up a geriatric unit there. 'Why?' I asked. 'What is your population over 65—two per cent?' 'I know', he replied, 'And its's growing all the time!' This is, I think, an eminently sensible, far-sighted attitude. In the West we are, in a sense, trying to shut the stable door when the horse has almost gone, and the attitude to those of us who are attempting the job is oddly ambivalent. Every week in the *British Medical Journal* at least one or two posts of consultant psychiatrist with a special interest in the elderly or even consultant psychogeriatrician is advertised, yet so far neither the Department of Health and Social Security nor even the Royal College of Psychiatrists accepts that the subspecialty actually exists. This is an important reason why it is hard to get a proper training in the art, and why candidates for the posts advertised are not infrequently not up to them. Critics claim that the specialty is only for administrative convenience, that it is too unattractive to draw enough people to do the work properly, and that as geriatrics is returning to general medicine psychogeriatrics should not break away from general psychiatry. I answer that there are special clinical skills involved, that the administrative aspects require a special knowledge, that the past record of general psychiatry in coping with the elderly is not all that impressive, that few general psychiatrists have the time or inclination to liaise adequately with geriatrics, that the field will become more attractive the better it is practised, taught and recognised, and that psychogeriatricians can still practice as general psychiatrists some but not most of the time, just as consultants in forensic and child psychiatry (both recognised subspecialties) may still do some general work.

At present the 100 or so psychogeriatricians in Britain mean that there is approximately one for every health district, or per half million population, not necessarily giving all his or her services to the elderly. The Section for the Psychiatry of Old Age considers that there should be at the least one whole time equivalent (which might mean two half timers) per quarter million population, so the number needs to be more than doubled very soon. Some general psychiatrists move over into geriatric psychiatry when there is no one else to do the job, and very welcome they are too. But for the young man or woman who wants a challenging and stimulating job the opportunities are immense, and the pioneering days are by no means over yet.

The importance of *liaison*, especially with geriatricians, local authorities and homes, has been emphasized repeatedly: it is essential for the best use of resources. How sensible, for instance, it would be if in every area, the psychogeriatric wards dealt with the most difficult, the geriatric with the most feeble and the residential homes with the remaining old people requiring institutional care without arguments about the exact criteria for each placement. Effective liaison requires not only good will and a sound knowledge of others' skills and resources, but the time for communication, which means not only finding time to talk, but choosing a time when the other can listen.

In the movement of psychiatric services from the mental to the district general hospitals it is most important that psychogeriatrics should not be left behind. Despite certain advantages in the design of mental hospital wards for old people (who are at least given plenty of leg room), the staffing problems once acute psychiatry has moved away will preclude effective care, and I see no future for the mental hospitals other than their ultimate closure. (One can imagine what picturesque ruins they will seem in two or three hundred years time, if all have not been totally demolished to make the sites available for housing.) Acute psychogeriatrics requires a ward to itself on the ground floor of the district psychiatric hospital's psychiatric department. In the same hospital, but as part of the geriatric department, should be a psychogeriatric assessment unit. Psychogeriatric patients requiring rehabilitation for up to one year should probably be accommodated in a second ward of the psychiatric department. Day patients may be distributed between the psychiatric and geriatric day hospitals (each attached to its own department) the more infirm going to the latter.

Longer-term psychogeriatric patients (the great majority demented) are supposed to be accommodated in community hospitals, i.e. those general hospitals which will not be upgraded to the district hospital standard, and which will be smaller, with less acute work. These will have the advantage for the psychogeriatric patient of being near to home, and it may be possible to find staff willing to work locally with confused old people from their own neighbourhood. However, unless rebuilt, the wards in most community hospitals will be too small and cramped for ambulant patients, and conditions could compre unfavourably even with the mental hospitals, let alone the residential homes.

With the development of EMI homes I wonder, indeed, if hospital is needed at all for the demented elderly whose behaviour, rather than phsyical health, is a problem. It is my impression that these homes are quite capable of coping with old people as residents who would be regarded as patients in a psychiatric hospital. Wandering, incontinence and even aggressiveness are not difficulties which obviously require hospital care. Perhaps the reasons the EMI homes do not already cope with all the demented elderly are firstly because there are not enough of them, and secondly because the hospitals are there. If the long-stay psychogeriatric wards were closed, then staff might be released who could work in the home. The situation is comparable with that of the subnormal, for whom the Department of Health hopes eventually to provide care solely in community homes. The arguments for and against EMI homes have been discussed in Chapter 18. Were there no dementia wards in psychiatric hospitals (which, of course, represent considerable segration), the arguments for integrated homes only might seem rather lame.

Costs must generally be counted. Homes are cheaper than hospital, and community care may be cheaper than homes. Some social workers in Kent were given less than the full cost of a place in a home to see if they could buy extra care for old people who would otherwise have taken that place and the experiment appeared to be a success both in the quality and duration of the old people's lives at home and financially. Hidden costs should, however, be considered too; that of drawing a full pension and supplements including rate rebates, for example. In Britain we are greatly committed to community care, and our institutions are not always very good. In some other countries there is a much greater committment to institutional care, some of a very high quality indeed. Is home always better than a home? I don't really think we know. The safest answer is that it is and it isn't.

Most countries, unless they produce an abundance of the black gold that is oil, cannot pay enough people to look after their elderly. It is therefore most important to make the public aware of the part they could and should play in the care of their older neighbours, whose ranks ere long they will join themselves.

Psychogeriatrics is an exciting new venture in psychiatry, rising to meet the challenge of mental disorder in the elderly rather than sidestep it. The effective practice of psychogeriatrics demands enthusiasm, energy, flexibility, patience, goodwill, honesty, diplomacy, a good knowledge of medicine, a thorough grounding in psychiatry, and an uncommon store of common sense. Few of us can lay claim to all these qualities, and I must confess that I am not infrequently as guilty of defeatism, domination, insularity and paranoia as the next three men. However, I hope that this book, however imperfect, arbitrary, inconsistent, opinionated or plain irritating it may be judged, will serve as a rough guide to a still largely undiscovered territory which remains to be more extensively explored in the years ahead.

REFERENCES

Arie T 1971 Morale and the planning of psychogeriatric services. Brit Med J 3: 166

Arie T, Isaacs A D 1978 The development of psychiatric services for the elderly in Britain. In Isaacs A D, Post F (eds) 'Studies in geriatric psychiatry'. Wiley, Chichester

Baker A A, Byrne R J F 1977 Another style of psychogeriatric service. Brit J Psychiat 130: 123

Godber C 1977 Conflict and collaboration between geriatric medicine and psychiatry. In Isaacs B (ed.) Recent advances in geriatric medicine. Churchill Livingstone, Edinburgh

Pitt B, Silver C P S 1980 The combined approach to geriatrics and psychiatry: evaluation of a joint unit in a teaching hospital district. Age and Ageing 9: 33

Appendix

SCHEME FOR PSYCHOGERIATRIC ASSESSMENT

Date

Patient's name, age, address, telephone number, GP and social worker.

Next of kin: name, age, address, telephone number, and relationship to patient.

Informant (if different): name, age, address, telephone number, and relationship to patient.

Reason for referral.

History of present condition (from patient and informant): the problem, its main features, how it began, how it has developed, whom it affects, how it has responded so far to treatment and management. For example, if the patient is confused, for how long? What were the circumstances at the onset? Has the course been intermittent, or steadily progressive? Any associated physical symptoms (blackouts, falls, paralysis)? Medication (could confusion be in part iatrogenic)? Wandering, getting lost, sleeplessness, fire-risk, leaving gas on, incontinence, aggression? Ability to shop, handle money, cook, do housework, dress and undress, wash and feed self? Is life endangered by self-neglect?

Past illness: physical and psychiatric. Any admissions to hospital? In last five years?

Family: age of parents at death, and what they died of? Father's occupation? How did parents get on? Size of family? Patient's place? Surviving brothers and sisters, where they live, and how much contact now? Where raised? Parental deprivation? Parent preferred? Was childhood home happy? Any unusual features of childhood? Has anyone in family suffered psychiatric illness? Details?

Personal history: schooling, and age of leaving school?

Main occupation? How long retired? Any current employment?

Men—any unemployment before 65, and why? Military service?

Current income and capital? Supplementary pension? Who collects pension?

Accommodation: nature, condition, rent (and whose is the rent-book), how long there, relations with neighbours? Reaction to any rehousing? Marriage: how often, and to whom? State of marriage? If widowed, for how long? Reaction to bereavement? Patient as spouse?

Children: where do they live? Address and telephone number? Frequency and quality of contact?

Patient as parent?

Previous personality and interests? Are any maintained? Drink and tobacco? How does patient fill day/week?

Social circumstances: whom does patient see in the course of a week? Clubs, Church, home help, Meals on Wheels, health visitor, district nurse, or any other professional or voluntary visitor?

Has any other specialist been consulted lately, or residential home been sought?

Examination: Physical (basic)—do nutrition and hydration seem adequate?

How well can patient see, hear and walk?

Any fever, hypothermia or heart failure? Plantar reflexes?

(Full physical examination for any patient admitted to hospital.)

Mental—orientation in time and place and for person: day, date, month, year, age, birthday, year of brith, present address, place of interview, recognition of family and friends? Queen, Royal Family, Prime Minister, President of the United States, current events, decimal currency (how many new pence in a pound, recognition of 50 p and 2 p pieces) and orientation. Ability to find bed, lavatory, kitchen. Ability to retain correct information when answers have been wrong? Speech: note any difficulty in finding right words (dysphasia), slurring (dysarthria), idiosyncratic use of words and phrases (metonyms—usually suggesting schizophrenia/paraphrenia).

If dysphasia or dyspraxia seem likely, ask patient to identify objects, obey simple commands, write name, copy drawn triangle.

Delusions, illusions, hallucinations? Details?

Mood—depressed, apathetic, elated, labile, irritable, suspicious, equable?

Insight—attitude to interrogation, awareness of disabilities and desire for help?

Appearance and manner—up or in bed, dressed or in dressing-gown, smart, shabby or soiled, cordial or hostile, confiding, or guarded? Relatives/friends—loving, concerned, ambivalent, indifferent, hostile, sincere or manipulative? What do they really want?

Home (if seen)—condition of garden, exterior, living room, kitchen, bedroom, bathroom (if any) and lavatory? Is home neat and clean, dingy and untidy, or frankly squalid? Is there enough food? (Are there empty bottles under the sink or in the dustbin?) Is there a lift (elevator)? Does it work? Is a car available? How near is a bus stop?

Diagnosis

Formulation

Possible actions
1. None needed
2. Advice on medication at home
3. Enlist more help from community services
4. Visit again
5. Refer to community psychogeriatric nurse
6. Follow up as outpatient
7. Treat as day patient
8. Recommend sheltered housing (old people's flat)
9. Recommend residential (old people's) home
10. Recommend admission to general or geriatric ward
11. Admit to psychogeriatric assessment unit
12. Admit to psychiatric ward.
    (Will admission directly help patient? If not, will it help key supporter, and is he/she sufficiently strained to need this help? Never openly admit for long-term care, only for assessment and treatment.)

SUGGESTED FURTHER READING

Some of these titles have already been listed at the end of chapters.

PSYCHOGERIATRICS

Arie T (ed.) 1981 Health care of the elderly. Croom Helm, London
Butler R N, Lewis M I 1977 Ageing and mental health: positive psychosocial approaches. Mosby, st Louis
Comfort A 1980 Practice of geriatric psychiatry. Elsevier, Holland
Howells J G 1975 Modern perspectives in the psychiatry of old age. Churchill Livingstone, Edinburgh
Isaacs A D, Post F 1979 Studies in geriatric psychiatry. Wiley, Chichester
Kay D W, Walk A (eds) 1971 Recent developments in psychogeriatrics. Brit J Psychiat, Special publication no 6. Headley, Ashford
Post F 1965 The clinical psychiatry of late life. Pergamon, London
Whitehead J M 1978 Psychiatric disorders in old age. Harvey Miller, London

AGEING AND THE OLD

Blythe R 1979 The view in winter. Allen Lane, London.
Bromley D B 1966 The psychology of human ageing. Harmondsworth: Penguin.
Carver V, Liddiard P 1978 An ageing population. Open University Press, Hodder and Stoughton, Sevenoaks
Care of the Elderly in Britain 1977 Central Office of Information, Pamphlet 121, H.M.S.O., London
Comfort A 1979 The biology of senescence. Elsevier, Holland
Comfort A 1977 A good age. Mitchell Beazley, London
Department of Health and Social Security 1978 A happier old age. H.M.S.O., London. Townsend, 1957. Wilmott and Young, 1960

DEMENTIA

Glen A I M, Whalley L J 1979 Alzheimer's disease. Churchill Livingstone, Edinburgh
Lishman W A 1977 Senile and presenile dementias. Medical Research Council, London
Lishman W A 1978 Organic psychiatry. Blackwell, London
Scottish Health Education Unit 1980 Forgetfulness and the elderly. How can you help? Edinburgh
Wells N E J 1979 Dementia in old age. Office of Health Economics, London

DEPRESSION

MacDonald A 1980 Depression and elderly people. Mind, London
Post F 1962 The significance of affective symptoms in old age. Maudsley Monography no. 10, Oxford University Press

PARANOID STATES

Post F 1966 Persistent persecutory states in the elderly. Pergamon, London

HEALTH IN OLD AGE

British Medical Journal 1974 Medicine in old age. Devonshire Press, Torquay
Coni N, Davison W, Webster S 1980 Lecture notes on geriatrics. Blackwell, Oxford
Hodkinson H M 1979 Common symptoms of disease in the elderly. Blackwell, Oxford, London
Isaacs B (ed.) 1978 Recent advances in geriatric medicine. Churchill Livingstone, Edinburgh

PSYCHOLOGICAL THERAPIES

Carr J 1980 Helping your handicapped child. Penguin, Harmondsworth
Holden U, Woods R 1982 Reality orientation therapy. Churchill Livingstone, Edinburgh
Parkes C M 1975 Bereavement: studies of grief in adult life. Penguin, Harmondsworth

DAY CARE

Peace S 1980 Caring from day to day: a report on the development of the day hospital within the service for elderly people who are mentally infirm. Mind, London

SOCIAL WORK WITH THE ELDERLY

Brearley C P 1979 A bibliography on social work and ageing. Age Concern, Mitcham
Glendenning F (ed) 1978 Social work with the elderly. Beth Johnson Foundation Publications, University of Keele
Gray B, Isaacs B 1979 Care of the elderly mentally infirm. Tavistock, London

SERVICE TO OLD PEOPLE

Department of Health and Social Security 1972 Services for mental illness related to old age. H.M. (72)71. H.M.S.O. London
Priorities for Health and Personal Social Services in England 1976 H.M.S.O., London
Enoch M D, Howells J (eds.) 1971 The organisation of psychogeriatrics. Society of Clinical Psychiatrists
Glasscote R, Gudeman J E, Miles D 1977 Creative mental health services for the elderly. Joint Information Service of the American Psychiatric Association and Mental Health Association, Washington D.C.

RESIDENTIAL CARE

Department of Health and Social Security 1977 Residential homes for the elderly: arrangements for health care. Welsh Office.
Townsend P 1962 The last refuge. Routledge and Kegan Paul
Wilkin D, Jolley D 1979 Behavioural problems among old people in geriatric wards, psychogeriatric wards and residential homes. Psychogeriatric Research Unit, Withington Hospital, Manchester

Index